Social Work

This is a tim ...nprecedented uncertainty and change in social work. However, as ...icture and organisation of services are in flux, the essential qu' ... social workers do not change – the ability to listen to people, to ... ...ate on behalf of others and to see people in the context of their whole ...es.

Social Wo *Voices from the inside* offers unique insight into social work from the ...nectives of those 'on the inside', that is, service users, carers and pra... ...rs. Drawing on a narrative tradition, 59 people from across the UK t ... stories about how and why social work came into their lives, and ... appened next. Topics covered include:

- children a..d ...ilies' social work
- criminal justic social work
- mental hea...h ocial work
- residentia' ...¹ care
- social wc ... disabled people
- social w... ... older people
- lessons f ... ...uture.

Focusing on ... ...r good practice in social work and social work educa-tion, this b(...sential reading for students and academics of social work and s... ...icy. It will also appeal to social work professionals and those in ...ealth, education and care areas.

Viviene E. C ...fessor of Social Work Studies in the School of Social & Poli... ...'ies at the University of Edinburgh.

Ann Davis is Professor of Social Work and Director of the Centre of Excellence in Interdisciplinary Mental Health at the University of Birmingham.

Social Work

Voices from the inside

Viviene E. Cree
and Ann Davis

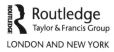

LONDON AND NEW YORK

First published 2007 by Routledge
2 Park Square, Milton Park, Abingdon, Oxon OX14 4RN

Simultaneously published in the USA and Canada
by Routledge
711 Third Avenue, New York, NY 10017

Routledge is an imprint of the Taylor & Francis Group, an informa business

© 2007 Viviene E. Cree and Ann Davis

Typeset in Times New Roman by
Florence Production Ltd, Stoodleigh, Devon

British Library Cataloguing in Publication Data
A catalogue record for this book is available from the British Library

Library of Congress Cataloging in Publication Data
   Social work: voices from the inside/Viviene E. Cree and Ann Davis.
       p. cm.
     Includes bibliographical references and index.
   1. Social work with women.   2. Women's health services – Social
   aspects.   3. Women – Social conditions.   4. Sexism in medicine.
   I. Cree, Viviene E., 1954–.   II. Davis, Ann.
   HV1444.S63 2006
   361.3–dc22   2006017654

ISBN10: 0–415–35682–2 (hbk)
ISBN10: 0–415–35683–0 (pbk)
ISBN10: 0–203–00283–0 (ebk)

ISBN13: 978–0–415–35682–4 (hbk)
ISBN13: 978–0–415–35683–1 (pbk)
ISBN13: 978–0–203–00283–4 (ebk)

Contents

Chapter 1

Voices from social work

INTRODUCTION

Our aim in writing this book is to present social work from the inside: from the perspectives of social work service users, carers and practitioners currently working and living with social work in the UK. It has been written at a time when across the four countries in the UK, social work is facing unprecedented uncertainty and change. On the one hand, social work is, for the first time, enjoying recognition of its standing alongside other professional groups. It is now a registered profession, with degree-level training. But social work is also experiencing high levels of insecurity and uncertainty. It is not at all clear where social workers are going to be employed and who will employ them in the future. In these new emerging structures and organisations, will social workers be replaced by other kinds of workers? And what will be the implications of this for those on the receiving end of services?

In the midst of this time of change, we invited a range of people to take stock: to help us to examine what people think they are delivering in the here and now, and what we might wish to take forward into the new world of social work. We therefore asked them to tell us about their journeys in and through social work practice. Whilst every story is unique, common themes emerge across the various accounts and, as authors, we have sought to contextualise these in the wider research literature so that readers may follow up the stories with further reading. Each contributor was invited to consider the positive part that social work might play in individual lives and in society as a whole, and these messages have been pulled together in the concluding chapter which provides an overview of the book.

A critical time for social work

The interviews for the book were conducted during 2005. This was a time when there were major consultations, discussions and debates about social work's role in the past, present and future, initiated by the Department of Health, the Social Care Institute for Excellence (SCIE), the National Assembly for Wales and the Scottish Executive. These debates reflect the New Labour government's 'Modernising' agenda, which has, at its heart, reform of the public sector. The overall aim of this has been expressed as 'putting people at the centre of public services' (Offices of Public Service Reform 2002); the underpinning belief is that services will become more effective 'if people are enabled to become participants in the design and delivery of services and so become co-producers of the public goods they value' (Leadbetter 2004). Of course, the drive to involve users of services has not simply been a government-inspired initiative. In recent years, carers, users of services and their organisations have led the way in challenging traditional paternalism in social work and health. Many of the recent developments in service delivery – for example, the shifts towards Direct Payments and Independent Living schemes – have come about as a direct result of campaigns by user groups (see Beresford and Croft 2004). Likewise, Davis (2006) and others have argued that service users and carers must in future be seen as active, knowledgeable agents, rather than passive recipients of services.

'Modernising' social services has not only been about user participation (see Cree 2002). It has, just as crucially, been concerned with breaking down the organisational barriers which existed between services, and creating 'new shared ways of delivering services that are individually tailored, accessible and more joined up' (Department of Health 2000: 30). The consequence for social work and social services in 2005 has been a whole-scale restructuring of service delivery and, with it, the demise of local authority social services and social work departments. As services for adults and children throughout the UK have become separated, so adult services are increasingly managed by departments of health, and children and family services by departments of education. These developments challenge the integrated nature of the social work profession and add to a sense of fragmentation and uncertainty. Questions have been asked about whether social work can survive in the new world. Whatever happens, the whole organisation and delivery of social work services in the future are set to look very different from social work in the past.

This was also a time of consolidation for social workers and the social work profession in the UK. After a long campaign waged over the last 25 years by professional bodies including the British Association of Social Workers (BASW) and the Central Council for Education and Training in Social Work (CCETSW), legislation was passed in 2000 and 2001 which regulated the social work profession for the first time. The Care Standards Act 2000 and Regulation of Care (Scotland) Act 2001 required that all qualified social workers should be registered. Social workers were invited to register from 1 April 2003; then from 1 April 2005 (England, Wales and Northern Ireland) and 1 September 2005 (Scotland), the title of social worker was protected for the first time, so that only those with an 'entitling qualification' could call themselves social workers. The registration of social workers will undoubtedly strengthen the profession, by giving social workers the same status as other professional groups such as teachers, nurses and doctors. It will also, it is hoped, act as a safeguard for users of services, and add to the general public's confidence in social work.

All of the changes we have highlighted demonstrate that this is a book of its time; it inevitably captures a moment – a moment when we know where we have come from, but cannot be certain where we are going. This does not suggest, however, that the fundamental social work practice which the book describes is likely to change quickly. On the contrary, the stories which the service users, carers and practitioners have shared with us are, in many ways, timeless, because it is clear that good practice in social work remains constant, while structures and organisations may change.

Some thoughts about terminology

It should be noted from the outset that the terms 'service user', 'carer' and 'practitioner' are all potentially unhelpful and may be misleading; the differences between these groups may, at times, be more apparent than real, as we will discover.

The term 'service user' has been used for a number of years in preference to the term 'client' as a convenient and neutral shorthand expression to denote those who are receiving social work services. However, many people who use services have not wished to be defined in this way, finding the term, at least, clumsy, and, at worst, derogatory and even oppressive. Those who use services are not a homogeneous group, as this book will demonstrate. They come from all classes and cultures; they are young and old, female and male, with disabilities and without. Neither are they only 'service users'; any one of us may need to access social services for a particular reason, but this is not our primary identity. What unites service users is that, for a time, they have individually (or as family members) accessed the services of social work. Some service user groups have introduced the term 'experts by experience' as a better way of defining their contribution (see Preston-Shoot 2005). We have continued to use the term 'service user' simply because it is more familiar in public usage.

The term 'carer' brings similar complications. From the 1960s onwards, there was an upsurge of interest in the notion of caring, reflecting wider political, social and economic changes that were taking place (Cree 2000). Social scientists and feminist researchers drew attention to the reality that what was being championed by successive governments as 'community care' was actually an unpaid and unseen domestic service performed largely by women. The 1980s therefore witnessed an explosion of concern for the experience of carers, at exactly the same time as disability rights campaigners instigated a movement for civil rights for people with disabilities. The consequence of both these developments has been the creation of a better understanding of the meaning of care, both to care-givers and to care-recipients. It has been acknowledged that caring is a complex, interconnected and changing experience in which people care for each other in different ways, at different times. What this implies for our own discussion is that the word 'carer' is not a straightforward, factual one. In practice, carers may also be cared for by those for whom they are caring, and the impact of class, gender, 'race'/ethnicity and other structured inequalities plays a major role in determining the quality and nature of that caring relationship.

We have argued that the terms 'service user' and 'carer' must not be taken at face value; neither should the term 'social worker'. We have already stated that 'social worker' is now a protected title in the UK. In writing this book, we have deliberately chosen the term 'social work practitioner' in preference to this, in order to acknowledge that there are many people practising in social work who are not called social workers. So, for example, the residential workers and leaving care team staff whom we interviewed are not called social workers. Nevertheless, the stories in this book are, with only one exception, the stories of those with professional social work qualifications who are working in different practice settings. Whilst we do not wish to minimise the contributions of the very many social work assistants, day-care staff and youth workers working in social services, this was not our primary focus in this book.

Terminology impacts on the contents of the book, as well as the titles of the contributors. Language is a hugely contested area, in social work as in other disciplines. Terms such as 'mental illness', 'disability' and 'offender' are highly emotive and will, at different points in time, carry different meanings and nuances. We have tried, wherever possible, to be sensitive to the language that service users and carers prefer to use to describe their experiences. This means that at times, language may be used which is no longer the preferred terminology within a professional group. One example of this is the word 'sectioned', which service users have used in their accounts to describe the experience of being hospitalised under mental health legislation.

There is one final point to be made here. In pulling together the accounts in the book, we have been struck by the reality that people's experiences are often overlapping and contradictory; their identities are not static, but are constantly changing. Hence someone who is, today, a service user, may train to become a social worker tomorrow; someone who is employed in social work may, at the same time, be a carer and possibly also a user of social services. This suggests that we must approach the book with some caution, and with a large measure of respect for the multi-layered, complex lives which people lead.

STRUCTURE OF THE BOOK

The book is structured around six broad areas of social work practice which are presented alphabetically:

- children and families' social work
- criminal justice social work
- mental health social work
- residential child care
- social work with disabled people
- social work with older people.

These areas reflect the reality of the organisation of social work practice in the UK to some degree, but they are not discrete categories. Nor do they constitute the only service user groups with whom social work is involved. There is, as is widely recognised, a large measure of overlap between social work with disabilities and mental health social work; likewise between mental health social work and social work with older people, particularly around the subject of dementia. At the same time, topics such as social work in the fields of addictions and youth justice have only received passing mention and deserve further consideration in the future. In writing the book, however, we had to start somewhere, and we believe that the range of work covered by these six broad areas allows the reader to build a reasonably accurate picture of social work as it is practised in the UK today.

The setting for the book, as stated, is social work in the UK. Interviews were conducted in Belfast, Cardiff, Edinburgh, Fife, London, the Midlands of England and Yorkshire. This is not to suggest that social work is the same across the UK; it is clearly not, as demonstrated by the inclusion of a chapter on criminal justice social work. We believe, however, that by taking readers into very specific examples of social work in different parts of the UK, we will give them access to more generalisable ideas about social work, and about its impact on service users, carers and practitioners wherever the setting.

CONTEXT OF THE BOOK

There is a rich mixture of material available which considers social work from the perspectives of service users, carers and practitioners.

Over the last 10 years or so, a number of edited books and anthologies of users' and carers' accounts have been published. For example, Read and Reynolds' (1996) collection provides a useful example of mental health service users' accounts of the services they had received, both in hospital and the community, and offers clear pointers as to what people want from mental health services in the future. More recently, Malone *et al.*'s (2005) anthology provides first-hand stories of how service users, carers and care professionals have experienced their everyday interactions, as well as examples of works of fiction which also provide another perspective on the issues raised.

The involvement of service users and carers cannot, Beresford and Croft argue, be understood in isolation:

> It needs to be understood in the much broader context of the development of movements of health and social care service users, including the disabled people's and mental health service users'/survivors' movements ... The focus of these movements has extended far beyond social work, social care and welfare into broader political, economic, social and cultural spheres.
>
> (2004: 62)

Recent SCIE reports (Social Care Institute for Excellence 2004a and 2004b) review the contribution that service user participation has made to social care services and to social work education. Whilst these reports identify that the involvement of service users and carers has been patchy, and is yet to be properly evaluated, nevertheless they demonstrate that participation is already challenging traditional professional modes of thinking and operating in a constructive way. As an example of this, the international journal *Social Work Education* invited an editorial collective of service users, carers and academics to produce a special issue dedicated to user involvement in social work education in 2006.

Just as there is current interest in service user and carer perspectives, so there has been renewed commitment to explore the experiences of those in the social care workforce. This has taken the form of both academic research and government review. Balloch *et al.*'s (1999) study of social workers in local authority social services departments uncovered evidence of high levels of stress and vulnerability to physical attacks. The study also, however, identified a relatively stable and committed workforce, which, on the whole, embraced change as offering positive opportunities and growth. Jones's (2001) research into social services department staff in England was less optimistic. He described the social workers whom he interviewed as stressed by their agencies, and social work as a 'factory through which people are processed'. More recently, Huxley *et al.* (2005) surveyed the stress and pressures experienced by mental health social workers and concluded that although the social workers in their study valued face-to-face contact with clients, they did not feel valued by their employers and society. This, they argue, is likely to lead to retention problems.

In contrast to this evidence of how social workers view their situation, a survey of public attitudes towards social work in Scotland found that the profession has a broadly positive profile (Davidson and King 2005). Of those who had used social work services, 78 per cent were said to be satisfied with the services they received and 69 per cent indicated that social services were quick to respond to their needs. Half of those surveyed agreed that they understood the role of social workers (37 per cent felt they did not understand the role) and 42 per cent of respondents had a positive or very positive perception of the work (with 24 per cent having a negative perception). Throughout the survey, research participants made references to staff shortages and there was recognition that social workers are required to undertake a wide range of difficult tasks and that some of the burden could be shifted to other agencies.

This more encouraging picture is also illustrated in the substantive reviews which have been undertaken in Scotland, England and Wales. In Scotland, *Changing Lives: the 21st Century Review of Social Work in Scotland*[1] draws attention to the reduction in the balance of time spent by social workers on developing therapeutic relationships with clients, yet these are identified as the areas most valued by the profession as a whole. The review also points out that local authority social workers and departments are risk-aversive and defensive in their decision-making, overly driven by processes, rather than outcomes. A similar review in England, conducted by the Commission for Social Care Inspectorate, published its first report in December 2005, entitled *The State of Social Care in England, 2004–05*.[2] This review highlights the positive difference which social care can make, but emphasises that people want, first and foremost, independence, choice and control in their lives, and to be treated with dignity. It also notes that the funding for social services is inadequate, leading to councils setting high thresholds for people to access services. Wales has also carried out a review of social work: *Social Work in Wales: A Profession to Value*.[3] This stresses the reality that it is not pay which is the driver in encouraging practitioners to remain in social work, but the culture of the organisation; this is therefore where improvement needs to take place.

Throughout this book, service users, carers and practitioners make reference to, and develop, many of the issues raised in this overview. In doing so, they are drawing on their direct and recent experience of social work practice 'from the inside'.

THEORETICAL CONTEXT

The book reflects and demonstrates the central idea that personal stories are a legitimate way of exploring and understanding the world. As Plummer writes:

> ... stories have recently moved centre stage in social thought. In anthropology, they are seen as the pathways to understanding culture. In psychology, they are the bases of identity. In history, they provide the tropes for making sense of the past. In psychoanalysis, they provide 'narrative truths' for analysis.
>
> (1995: 18)

Anglo-American social work has been slow to take up a narrative approach. Fraser argues that narrative approaches, 'with the capacity to recognise people's strengths and engage people in active, meaning-making dialogues', have much to offer the discipline of social work (2004: 181).

While social work practice may have been slow to adopt narrative ideas, researchers and activists have increasingly made use of biographical and autobiographical approaches to tell stories of the unheard voices in social work: disabled people, older people, survivors of sexual abuse, looked-after children and others. What these studies have in common is a shared understanding of the validity of the accounts of the storytellers: an acceptance of the idea that we all tell stories of our lives, and that these stories constitute knowledge, just as much as any more so-called 'scientific' approach to research. Foucault asserts that rediscovery of 'indigenous' or 'local popular' knowledge holds the key to bringing about change:

> I also believe that it is through the re-emergence of these low-ranking knowledges, these unqualified, even directly disqualified knowledges ... which involve what I would call a popular knowledge ... that criticism performs its work.
>
> (1980: 82)

This suggests that an approach which builds on individuals' stories is not only a useful research device, but also potentially transformative.

The narrative turn builds on the oral history and life history tradition. Since the 1960s and 1970s, historians have been engaged in capturing the histories of people who have been ignored by history: working-class people, women, rural workers, older people, gay and lesbian people (see Denzin 1989, Plummer 2001, Thompson 2000). Linda Gordon's (1988) history of family violence in Boston, Massachusetts, between 1880 and 1860 is called *Heroes of Their Own Lives*. Her book title captures extremely well how we feel about the people who have contributed to this book.

Our book is a follow-up to *Becoming a Social Worker*, edited by Cree (Routledge 2003). *Becoming a Social Worker* relates the accounts of those who work in social work: social work students, academics and practitioners from different social work settings across the UK. Thirteen people were invited to reflect on and write about their decisions to enter the social work profession, and their career progression from that point on. The book provided surprising and illuminating stories about social work and social workers – what they thought about social work, and what they thought about themselves in relation to social work. This led to the idea to take this exercise in autobiography one step further, by exploring the similar and different stories of service users, carers and practitioners.

Unlike the earlier book, this is not an edited collection. Nor is it an illustration of empirical research findings; instead, it lies somewhere in between. Drawing on a narrative research/life history tradition, we encouraged people to tell us their stories – of their lives and of social work – so that we could learn from their understandings of their experiences and interactions in their lives. Each chapter presents the stories passed on to us through interviews with 59 service users, carers and practitioners across the UK.

METHODOLOGY

Interviews were set up with the support and facilitation of social work academics and practitioners in the different parts of the UK. These 'gatekeepers' recommended people whom they knew and contacted them on our behalf (see Sutton 2004). We then followed up this initial contact and set up meetings. Many of the contributors then went on to recommend others for us to meet, in the convention of 'snowball' sampling, widely recognised as a helpful technique for gaining access to hidden or hard-to-reach populations (Atkinson and Flint 2001).

The decisions taken about how to access likely contributors inevitably had an impact on our findings. Most fundamentally, it seems reasonable to suggest that those who were recommended by others probably characterise those with more positive stories to tell. Moreover, those who then agreed to be interviewed were those who had something to say; they had learned something about social work or at least they had an idea about how they would like to see social work improved in the future. We do not, however, see this as a problem. This book is not a research study, and our contributors are not, and we do not make claim for them to be, representative of social work service users, carers or practitioners. Given the breadth and depth of subjects we have covered, they can be seen only to offer a taste of social work practice across the different fields and geographical areas.

Although this was not strictly a research study, our proposals were reviewed by the University of Edinburgh's School of Social & Political Studies Research Ethics Committee as a safeguard for ourselves and for the contributors. All of the interviews were tape-recorded and transcribed by the authors. The contributors received written information in advance, explaining the purpose and content of the interview and inviting them to take part in the book project. They were then asked to sign a consent form at the start of the interview. Contributors were offered expenses for taking part, as well as copies of audiotapes or transcripts of interviews; they also received copies of the book itself. In conducting the interviews, there were issues of confidentiality around the naming of individuals: contributors, their family members, practitioners, colleagues and managers. These issues were discussed, and contributors were invited to provide a pseudonym for themselves and others, if they wished to do so.

Our interview schedule was deliberately open. We were interested in setting broad parameters which would enable contributors to share with us the stories which *they* found most relevant. We also set out to ask them to share one event or incident which crystallised for them their experience of social work (see Fook 2002).

Service users and carers were asked about:

- You and why social work came into your life
- The kind of help you have received over the years
- An event that stands out for you as a time when social work really made a difference in your life (a 'critical incident')
- What you consider are important lessons for social workers in the future.

In parallel, social workers were asked about:

- You and why you decided to become a social worker
- Your career history – the work you have done over the years
- An event that stands out for you as a time when social work really made a difference (a 'critical incident')
- What you consider are important lessons for social workers in the future.

All the contributors came to the interviews with stories to tell, and sometimes also with curricula vitae and educational and work-related certificates to share with us as well. The request to share a critical incident resulted in many of them doing considerable reflection in advance of the interview and, for some, life review. Listening to the taped interviews in the quiet of our homes reminded us over and over again that we, in practice, often needed to say very little in the course of the interviews, except to add an occasional 'uh-huh' or perhaps to share a story from our own social work lives, to make a connection with what was being said.

This raises an interesting issue about truth and validity: how do we know that our contributors were telling us 'the truth'? It is a well-known fact of social science research that informants will seek to present themselves in a positive light (Mishler 1986). Moreover, human memory is fallible, and forgetting and distortion increase over time (Baddeley 1979). Our view is that neither of these seeming 'problems' takes away from the usefulness of the accounts which were shared with us; on the contrary, they can be seen as adding to the overall picture, since in retelling their stories, informants inevitably shared with us their current constructions of themselves, their lives and their interactions with others in the present and in the past. It was evident in listening to the contributors that some stories had been told and retold so many times that any inconsistencies and confusions had been ironed out along the way. Other stories came out in a rush, perhaps when a question triggered an answer which had not been voiced aloud before. In both instances, the stories were inevitably constrained by the events of a life (Bruner 1990); they were also shaped by the artificial nature of the encounter between the contributor and ourselves, as is the case in all social research. None of this makes the stories any less 'true'; on the contrary, it adds to the depth of understanding which these accounts bring.

It is also important to state that the accounts we received were not usually whole stories, with a clear beginning, middle and end. What we heard (and therefore relate in the book) were parts of a jigsaw; sometimes contributors may not themselves have been in a position to fill in the empty pieces. For example, one of the 'looked-after' young people who spoke to us did not know exactly why she had been taken into care, aged 4 years. There were times during interviews when we deliberately did not encourage the narrator to talk about a particularly difficult or painful time in her or his life. We were conscious that for all the contributors, this was a one-off interview, and that we did not know enough about the person's life to be sure that he or she would receive support, if required, after the interview. (We did, however, discuss this with our 'gatekeepers' on a number of instances.) Moreover, we knew this was not a counselling interview, and we were not, in this situation, social workers. We therefore sought to be attentive and open to contributors' stories, but at the same time respect their privacy, and not press them down avenues we felt they did not wish to go down (see Birch and Miller 2000).

Whilst we have edited and organised the accounts, we have sought, as much as possible, to allow the 'voices' to speak for themselves. This means that we have not made any attempt to assess the effectiveness of the social work practice being described. Nor have we suggested that one form of intervention is more or less useful than other. Instead, we have allowed any judgement of usefulness to rest with the narrator, that is, with the service user, carer or practitioner who is describing the work. Hence we do not get into debate about whether mental health services can or should 'cure' mental illness, just as any discussion about whether criminal justice social work can reduce offending remains an open question. But, by picking up and developing ideas from contributors, the conclusion suggests some lessons for the future.

The process of conducting the interviews and gathering the stories together into coherent chapters has been enlightening for us as authors and as social workers. We have found our passion for social work rekindled, and we have felt awed by the commitment that practitioners bring to their working lives. We have also been made acutely aware of how service users and carers are actively involved in working to ensure that the services they receive meet their needs, when they need them. Encouraging others to reflect on social work has forced us to rethink some of our views and experiences, and this self-reflection (reflexivity) has allowed us to think about where we currently sit on the journey from service user to carer to practitioner and back again (see Hertz 1997). The book also introduced us to a whole new set of friendships, with each other and with the contributors, and this has enriched the eventual product greatly.

LOOKING AHEAD

We have said in this chapter that we do not know what the organisation of social work services will look like in the future. But we have argued that the necessary qualities of social workers do not change: their ability to listen to people, to advocate on behalf of others and see them in the context of their whole lives. These are the qualities which stand out in social work, and are demonstrated throughout the stories in this book.

Shotter (1993) asserts that to be our social selves, to be individuals functioning within social and political communities, we need to 'voice' our identities and so participate in the active reproduction of these communities. This book seeks to ground social work practice in the real experiences of those who receive and deliver services so that we might reclaim our social work community. In doing so, we hope that readers might be encouraged to rethink the idea of social work practice as a partnership between the service user, carer and practitioner, where each may recognise the role and input of the other, and work together to improve services for the good of all.

NOTES

1 See www.21csocialwork.org.uk
2 See www.csci.gov.uk/publications
3 See www.allwalesunit.gov.uk

REFERENCES

Atkinson, R. and Flint, J. (2001) 'Accessing Hidden and Hard-to-reach Populations: Snowball Research Strategies', *Social Research Update*, Guildford, Surrey: University of Surrey.

Balloch, S., McLean, J. and Fisher, M. (1999) *Social Services: Working under Pressure*, Bristol: Policy Press.

Baddeley, A. (1979) 'The Limitations of Human Memory: Implications for the Design of Retrospective Surveys', from Moss, L. and Goldstein, H. (eds) *The Recall Method in Social Surveys*, London: University of London Institute of Education.

Beresford, P. and Croft, S. (2004) 'Service Users and Practitioners Reunited: the Key Component for Social Work Reform', *British Journal of Social Work*, 34: 53–68.

Birch, M. and Miller, T. (2000) 'Inviting Intimacy: the Interview as Therapeutic Opportunity', *International Journal of Social Science Methodology*, 3(3): 189–202.

Bruner, J. (1990) *Acts of Meaning*, Cambridge, MA: Harvard University Press.

Cree, V.E. (2002) 'The Changing Nature of Social Work', in Adams, R., Dominelli, L. and Payne, M. (eds) *Social Work. Themes, Issues and Critical Debates*, Basingstoke, Hants: Palgrave, pp. 20–9.

Davidson, S. and King, S. (2005) *Public Knowledge of and Attitudes to Social Work in Scotland*, Edinburgh: Scottish Executive Social Research.

Davis, A. (forthcoming 2006) 'Social Work in Europe: Building Credibility through Inclusionary Practice, a View from the UK', in Roloff, G. (ed.) *Contributions of the Human Sciences to a Fairer Practice*, Berlin: Pabst Science Publishers.

Denzin, N. (1989) *Interpretive Biography*, London: Sage.

Department of Health (2000) *A Quality Strategy for Social Care*, London: DoH.

Fook, J. (2002) *Social Work. Critical Theory and Practice*, London: Sage.

Foucault, M. (1980) *Power/Knowledge. Selected Interviews and Other Writings*, New York: Pantheon Books.

Fraser, H. (2004) 'Doing Narrative Research. Analysing Personal Stories Line by Line', *Qualitative Social Work*, 3(2): 179–201.

General Social Care Council/Social Care Institute for Excellence (2004) *Living and Working Together Conference Report*, London: GSCC and SCIE.

Gordon, L. (1988) *Heroes of Their Own Lives*, New York: Viking.

Hertz, R. (ed.) (1997) *Reflexivity and Voice*, London: Sage.

Huxley, P., Evans, S., Gately, C., Webber, M., Mears, A., Pajak, S., Kendall, T., Medina, J. and Katona, C. (2005) 'Stress and Pressures in Mental Health Social Work: the Worker Speaks', *British Journal of Social* Work, 35(7): 1063–80.

Jones, C. (2001) 'Voices from the Front Line: State Social Workers and New Labour', *British Journal of Social Work*, 31: 547–62.

Leadbetter, C. (2004) *Personalisation through Participation*, London: Demos.

Malone, C., Forbat, L., Robb, M. and Seden, J. (eds) (2005) *Relating Experience. Stories from Health and Social Care*, London: Routledge.

Mishler, E.G. (1986) *Research Interviewing. Context and Narrative*, Cambridge, MA: Harvard University Press.

Offices of Public Service Reform (2002) *Reforming Our Public Services*, London: OPSR.

Plummer, K. (1995) *Telling Sexual Stories: Power, Change and Social Worlds*, London: Routledge.

—— *Documents of Life 2: An Invitation to Critical Humanism*, London: Sage.

Preston-Shoot, M. (2005) 'Editorial', *Social Work Education*, 24(6): 601–02.

Read, J. and Reynolds, J. (eds) (1996) *Speaking Our Minds: An Anthology*, Basingstoke, Hants: Macmillan.

Shotter, J. (1993) 'Becoming Someone: Identity and Belonging', in Coupland, N. and Nussbaum, J.F. (eds) *Discourse and Lifespan Identity*, Newbury Park, CA: Sage.

Social Care Institute for Excellence (2004a) *Involving Service Users and Carers in Social Work Education*, Resource Guide no. 2, London: SCIE.

—— (2004b) *Has Service User Participation Made a Difference to Social Care Services?* Position Paper no. 3, London: SCIE.

Sutton, C.D. (2004) *Social Research: the Basics*, London: Sage.

Thompson, P. (2000) *The Voice of the Past. Oral History*, 3rd edition, Oxford: Oxford University Press.

Chapter 2

Children and families' social work

INTRODUCTION

Social work with children and families spans a wide range of activities directed at protecting children, promoting their well-being and working to support children to live with their families. It occupies a contested territory where the state intervenes in family life (Featherstone 2004). It is an area of social work which has received a great deal of, often hostile, media attention, focused on a succession of inquiries which have found that social workers, amongst others, have failed to keep children safe (see Butler and Drakeford 2005, Laming 2003). In recent years, children and family services have been subject to a series of policy and organisational changes, framed by major pieces of legislation across the UK (for example, the 1989 and 2004 Children Acts in England and Wales) and key policy documents (for example, Department for Education and Skills 2003, Department of Health and Department for Education and Skills 2004, Secretary of State for Health 2003). These have constructed a role for social workers which combines contributing to the assessment of the needs of children and young people, protecting them from harm and consulting and working with other relevant agencies, such as housing, education and health, to deliver services that promote children's well-being and safety in partnership with them and their families.

The organisational base for social work with children and families is shifting too, from a mix of individual specialist statutory and voluntary children and family social work organisations. In England, children's trusts have been created to integrate social work, education and health services through multi-agency working from a range of community-based locations. These changes are being promoted as offering social workers new ways of working collaboratively with other children and family professionals, ways that contrast with the limited, reactive roles which have characterised statutory children and family social work services (Garrett 2003). The changes which are currently reframing social work in this area claim to have, at heart, the interests of children and families and to be working for their involvement. Yet evidence suggests that despite these changes, 'families continue to struggle to access services before a crisis occurs, and collaboration between professional and service users continues to be a challenge' (Morris 2005: 75).

Whilst social work with children and families is focused on keeping children in their birth families, this is not always possible. It is estimated that 80,000 children in England in any one year are looked after outside of their birth families (Department for Education and Skills 2003). Two-thirds of these children are placed with foster-parents. The needs they present, as well as their continuing contact with their own families, have made fostering an increasingly challenging area of children and families' work for both social workers and foster-parents. In reviewing research evidence on children's experiences of foster-care, Sinclair (2005) argues that, to date, the organisation of fostering services in the UK has failed to give foster-parents the resources they need to make a coherent contribution to the ongoing lives of the majority of fostered children. The *Every Child Matters* agenda, in acknowledging poor outcomes for these children and young people in England, has set key targets for services in relation to achieving placement stability as well as improved educational outcomes for this group in the future (Department for Education and Skills 2003).

THE CONTRIBUTORS

Fourteen people contributed to this chapter. Thirteen live and work in the English Midlands, the 14th, a social worker, works in Yorkshire. Some of the service users and carers had contact with social workers because they were parents who found themselves in difficulties; others were foster-parents. The social work practitioners had accumulated a wealth of experience in children and family services spanning crisis/duty work; fostering and adoption services; and therapeutic work. All are women, many are parents themselves and their stories suggest that their contributions to the services employing them draw on a commitment to fight injustice, protect the vulnerable and promote family life in its diverse forms.

Service users and carers

David and Pauline

David said: 'I am 55 and have a partner and two children. One was born to us and the other was placed with us for adoption 7 years ago. I have worked as a social worker and am now a lecturer in social work. So it's been quite a sea change being on one side of the fence and then experiencing being a consumer on the other side.'

Pauline said: 'I am 53 and have a partner and two children, one was born to us and the other is placed with us for adoption. I have worked as a social worker in social services and voluntary organisations. Currently I am a Children's Guardian.'[1]

Jason

I am a single dad with two kids, a son and a daughter. The most important thing in my life is being there for my kids. I have been working as a warehouseman but I was recently made redundant.

Julie

I am a single mother of two children. I don't work, I am a sociable person, very easy-going but I have my problems like everyone else. I have a few friends and if I can help someone I will. I just do my day-to-day motherhood thing and try my best at everything and I'm not scared to ask for help if I need it. I am on my own with my kids and I'm pretty happy with the way things are.

Matt

I'm a manager in a local supermarket. I have always lived in the same area, never wanted to move away. I am divorced with two daughters who came to live with me a couple of years ago. I am a keen football fan and I play in a local league. I'm getting a bit old for playing now so I'm training to be a referee.

Practitioners

Barbara

I was the eldest daughter in my family and cared for my mother who was disabled. I went into further education late in life and became a social worker 11 years ago. I have been married for 45 years, all my children are in professional jobs and I have four grandchildren and four step-grandchildren.

Ellen

I think I am a very secure person, I think I have learnt to live with my good bits and the not so good bits and I feel quite well rounded and comfortable with myself. I love my family and we are a very close network, so they are very important to me.

Jan

I think I would describe myself as a social worker through and through, like a stick of rock really. Good with people, good sense of humour, generally optimistic.

Kuldeep

I am a single parent with two children. I came to England from India when I was young but have lived in England for most of my life.

Margaret

I'm a therapeutic social worker and I enjoy being in a position where I listen to people.

Sheila

I am in my early 40s, a white British woman. I have lived here all my life. I have been in social work in some form or another for 20 years since I left university. I have moved around the country a lot, I have changed direction, have married and had children, but I am still here in social work.

Sue

I have had a career in social work since 1971. Apart from that I am a wife and I have two adult children. I have tried to manage both sides of my life as effectively as I could. I didn't work full-time after I had the children because I felt it was important I should be there for them. My husband is also a social worker and I don't think it's fair on children having two parents full-time in social work.

Trish

I'm single with no children and glad about that. Since starting social work at a senior level, I have put off having them. I think I am friendly, sociable, and a hard worker. I like to sing. I learnt to play guitar a couple of years ago which means I now smoke like a sparrow because my hands are busy.

Vicky

I'm 35 years old, and I live quite locally to the area that I work in. I came into social work in 1996 and prior to that I worked with horses –

I had no connection with social work at all. I'm doing an MA in Child Protection and Child Welfare just now at the University of Huddersfield. It's a 3-year, part-time course, and I'm in my last year.

EXPERIENCING PARENTING

Julie and Jason first met social workers as a result of troubles in their lives as parents. As Julie explains:

> I was living with a partner who was a heroin addict and two children. It was quite hard because I had money robbed. There were lies and I had to deal with the children knowing. My oldest girl was 14 then and she knew something was going on. Then the inevitable happened and I started taking drugs. My daughter knew this and she started rebelling and getting aggressive with me and hitting me. My son, who was 6 then, started seeing a lot of violence. All of a sudden, my nice home started becoming a punch-up – a place where children were hitting me and I was trying to hide my drugs. So I called the police on my daughter – it was getting really bad.

The police put Julie in touch with social services and two social workers came to visit her. She asked them for respite care for her daughter, so that she could have some space to sort things out for the family. After several interviews with her and her daughter, the social workers asked them to attend a case conference to talk about the future:

> They said it was to discuss things, but it was full of strangers and I didn't feel good in it. They used words I didn't understand and talked about me, not to me. Then afterwards they gave my daughter ongoing counselling and a social worker came out to see me and my son to check my house again. He came out and I broke down and told him everything, but he seemed to think things were OK and he signed me off their books and that was that.

Julie's daughter went to live with her grandmother, and 8 months later, Julie was contacted by a family centre run by a local voluntary organisation. The referral had been made by social services and Julie said she welcomed it because she had ongoing problems – her partner had left and she found herself alone with parenting responsibilities. From the start, she found contact with the centre's social worker a positive experience:

> A social worker introduced herself to me, said who had referred me and gave a brief description about what she had been told had been

going on. There was nothing about my drugs, they hadn't mentioned it. She asked me if I would like a visit. I said I would. I was a bit defensive at first; I felt I was being checked on about my parenting. A couple of weeks later, I was introduced to the social worker I still have. My social worker still deals with my daughter but she focuses on me and my son and what is happening to us. She wants to keep us together and it is much more personal about what is happening in my home and it's about helping me.

Jason's contact with social workers began unexpectedly when his son was admitted to hospital:

Social work came into my life about 9 years ago. It was when my son was 1. The doctors told us he had a bleed at the back of his eyes. We took him to the hospital and it was a week and a half before the doctors actually told us what was wrong. We kept asking and asking but they said they wouldn't tell us nothing. They said it was a bleed on the brain and that it was basically down to shaking. They said someone must have shook him. I was accused of doing it before they asked us any questions. It was a matter of, 'It's the husband or boyfriend', it always is, the first time isn't it? I was arrested for it – charged with grievous bodily harm against my child.

Then they started to question us. There were case conferences, interviews, meetings, talking to social workers. Then they thought it was the mother – the suspicion fell onto her. The way they told us was they had got all this information together and they put it into the computer and the computer said the baby had been shaken. When this was happening, I didn't sleep for 5 days. I didn't eat; I lost nearly 2 stone [12.7 kg] in weight. I was just worn out emotionally and kept crying all the time for no reason – it was a real bad time.

It was recommended that Jason and his partner move with their children into a residential centre where their parenting skills would be assessed. In Jason's view, there was no choice:

They put us in the centre for a year, to watch us and the way we were with the kids. The social workers said they were giving us a choice. The choice was basically we could go to the centre and live there as a family to be assessed. They said if we didn't go we would lose the kids. It wasn't a choice really. If you wanted to keep your kids you had to go. The centre has self-contained flats and these flats are occupied with different families from all over the country. You are in there and they assess how you are looking after your kids. They come and see you and watch how you are bathing the baby and how you are feeding the baby and they write down things and sit and watch you and you have got to put up with it. If you want to keep your kids you have to do it.

During his time at the centre, Jason was involved in regular case conferences to discuss progress and the future. Like Julie, he found it difficult to take part in these meetings. Although Jason and his family expected to stay in the centre for only 3 months, they ended up staying for a year, because of rent arrears which meant that they could not return to local authority housing:

I said to social services, 'Why not give us a loan? If you pay for my rent arrears we could be out of this place.' But the council wouldn't give me a house, because of the arrears and because social services wouldn't pay them off to the council. In the end, we had to take the council to court and I only got a house then because my two kids have got disabilities. My son has a mild form of cerebral palsy and my daughter was born with one arm that stops at the elbow. In court, the judge said he was disgusted at the social services and the housing manager for not finding us a property. It meant that we had been in the centre for a year and he said we needed to get back in the community and he was right. It was the next day, after the court hearing, that we were offered this house.

Jason's partner left soon afterwards and he gave up work to look after the children. He had no furniture and no income for several months, because the social security and child benefit offices he contacted to establish his entitlement found it difficult to accept that he had become a lone parent. UK research evidence demonstrates that poverty experienced by families with children increases dramatically when parents are unemployed (see Joseph Rowntree Foundation 2005). This is compounded when, as in Jason's situation, lone parenthood and being a member of an ethnic minority are part of the equation. The impact of poverty, as well as poor housing in disadvantaged communities, has been identified as a major component of social exclusion, having a marked impact not only on the health and well-being of children, but also on their life chances (Preston 2005). Services directed at the protection and well-being of children, including social work, need to recognise and address these issues when working to support parents in difficulties (Davis and Wainwright 2005).

For Matt, David and Pauline, contact with social workers was made because they decided to open up their family homes to other children. David and Pauline had one son and decided to extend their family through adoption. Matt, in his early 20s with two young daughters and a partner who was a child-minder, felt he was talked into it:

It was through the child-minding that Kath heard about fostering for social services. I wasn't keen. To be honest, I was knackered – working long hours with the supermarket. Two kids seemed enough but she nagged me about it. I remember the first meeting we went to. They talked about what fostering involved and talked about why some kids needed it. It opened my eyes, it was a new world to me. It know it sounds terrible, but I hadn't really thought about what happens when kids don't have the homes they should – parents who are ill, drug addicts, violent. It was an eye-opener.

Both couples went to training sessions as part of the preparation and selection processes. For Matt, the training offered opened up new horizons not just in relation to understanding what was happening to children in need but in relation to his own attitudes and behaviour:

When I went to the classes, I was a bit stroppy – going back to the classroom – I never got on at school. But it wasn't like that – we had to talk things through in groups; say what we thought, how we would react, and we were challenged about what we said. It wasn't easy. There was a session about being racist – I thought it was well out of order. My school was full of Asians and West Indians, I got on OK with everyone – but they made me think – think about what I said and how I behaved. By the end of it, both of us were really keen and they seemed to think we might make a go of fostering.

Given David's and Pauline's own social work backgrounds, they were already familiar with the processes involved in becoming adoptive parents, but they were surprised by their reactions to being on the receiving end. David said that the actual assessment procedure had been a validating experience. However, he and Pauline both had reservations about the 3-day training programme which they thought was rather bland and promotional and did not, in Pauline's view, 'help people really consider some of the issues that they would have to think about, on a practical day-to-day level'.

A 3-year-old boy, Danny, was placed with them for adoption soon after the assessment process was completed. They found their lives transformed. Their parenting experiences in relation to their birth son, Tom, had not prepared them for the new addition to their family. They found Danny needy, disruptive and 'unreachable' and they were struggling. But they felt unable to be completely open about this with the social workers because, in Pauline's words, 'if we had laid it on the line about what he was really like and how hard we found it to live with him, they would remove him – and God help him then'.

David and Pauline struggled to get therapeutic help for Danny. They eventually secured the help of a psychotherapist for themselves and Danny, but they felt that the children and families' social workers who were in contact with them over this period were unsupportive and critical of their parenting. This response contrasted markedly with the support given to them by the adoption support social worker who visited and offered guidance. Pauline, in particular, found her presence helpful: 'It must have been difficult for her to take all my pain, because when I started talking, I'd just cry and cry and she would sit there through that with me.' David and Pauline have continued to provide a home for Danny who is now 10. But they are clear that they will not go for an adoption order until they get the back-up they need to meet his ongoing emotional and behavioural needs. They have learnt how difficult it is to get social work, mental health and educational services to focus on an individual child and work in partnership to make an appropriate response to his needs as well as those of his birth and adoptive families.

Matt and his partner decided to become short-term, respite foster-parents and he remembers warmly the social worker they worked with initially:

> Our first social worker was a gem of a woman. Maureen, I felt that she was interested in us and the girls as well as the children she was working with – a good listener, nothing fazed her; solid through and through. I felt we could share anything with her and it would be OK – she wouldn't judge us and would always find a way through.

When Maureen moved away to work for another local authority, he and his partner had a succession of social workers, some of whom seemed unfamiliar with fostering procedures, and some, he felt, seemed tired and overwhelmed with their workloads. The support they received was intermittent but the problems they were facing were constant. It was difficult to 'keep on top of' the procedures and paperwork involved with short-term fostering. There were also times when they found themselves with major difficulties trying to manage the parenting of their birth children alongside their fostered children. In desperation, they turned again to Maureen who had left her phone number with them and they were grateful that she took time to give them advice and guidance. When Matt's partner decided to end their marriage, it was Maureen who again provided a listening ear as Matt sorted out what to do about the care of his daughters as well as the foster-children that they were caring for.

WHAT HELPS?

The varied accounts of social work related by the service users reflect a mix of positive and negative experiences. Yet across this range, common themes emerged about what social work can do to help families in difficulties.

Listening and making judgements

Julie's recollections of her first contact with social workers were that they made assumptions about her as a drug user and an inadequate mother. Their actions (checking her house and cupboards to see if she was making provision for her children) as well as their words conveyed to her that they thought she couldn't parent and this framed her ongoing contacts with them. In contrast, from the outset, her current social worker established her concern to work with Julie on the issues that she identified as important. No judgements were made and no questions asked about her past, Julie shared what she wanted to when she was ready. It was this approach that Julie thought had helped her:

> I look at the future in a different way. My social worker has helped me find myself and I know where I am going now. Without her, I wouldn't know where I was, I would still have been in a mess somewhere. But I feel confident now about my future and I know now I can look after my son and that I am a good mum and I can do it – that's what she's shown me.

Jason, thinking about his experiences, had a clear message for all social workers working with families where the abuse of children is an issue:

> You need to listen to people and not judge them. In a lot of cases it is the boyfriend or husband who's the problem. But social workers shouldn't presume that at the start, they shouldn't start there, it could be different to that. You need to find out about the individual first.

Pauline, David and Matt recognised that being judged was part of the assessment, recruitment and training processes that they had to go through to become foster and adoptive parents. Indeed for all of them, being judged as people with a lot to give to children was a positive experience. However, when they fostered they found they needed a listening ear to share the problems they were facing as parents. Without this response, they not only felt unsupported, they felt they could not make full use of what they had to offer as foster-parents. As Matt saw it, the succession of social workers who had contact with them over the years 'talked about working together but it never really felt like that. We just seemed to be there to do the caring when they decided – on their terms. We were just a port in the storm – no more than that.'

Establishing relationships

Where social workers had been successful in establishing relationships, service users felt that they were able to be open and honest about what was happening to them. Matt and Julie described some very positive experiences of two social workers who were there for them. They had felt confident about sharing their difficulties openly with them and they described the way they had learnt from these relationships how to make difficult decisions about their futures as parents and people. When Matt thought about their first social worker who had kept in touch with them he recalled: 'She seemed to be able to tune in, listen and show us a way – she never lost touch. I don't know what we would have done without her. Knowing she was there for us.'

David, Pauline and Jason had had very different experiences. In the turmoil and difficulties facing them, they had to relate to a range of individuals who did not always build the kind of relationships that they could use to address the issues facing them. In reflecting on his experiences, David said:

> What I cannot get over is just how much a service and a response from that service is dependent on the individual professional, the face of the social services *is* that person and the relationship you have with that person and the judgements they make of you. If you fall out with them, or they don't see the world the way you do, as a service recipient, you can be in real trouble.

Reliable and responsive

All the contributors described incidents in their lives when they felt they were in crisis as parents and they needed a response from a social worker. Julie's social worker has given her what she needed:

> With my social worker there have been times when I have been on my own and been at loggerheads with myself when my children have been really getting me down and I have been able to pick the phone up to her and tell her what's happening and she hasn't judged me. She's talked me through things on the phone and if needed she's come straight out to deal with the situation there and then. She can't obviously come out all the time, but her words of wisdom over the phone have been there for me.

Jason made the point that support needed to be about more than just emotional or listening support – it needed to be practical too. When he was living in a house without any furniture and had no social security benefits to live on, he phoned up the social worker who had been allocated to him:

> I phoned him up and said, 'Look, man, I've got no food in the house, I'm still getting no money from the social, there's no food here, I don't know where you are, I've got to go out and shoplift, I'm starving and the kids are starving.' So he came up later in the day and given me some money a section 17 payment.[2] I had to threaten that twice to get some help from him. They gave me £30 each time and that's the only financial assistance they offered. It wasn't right – I just wasn't supported. It was written down, we had a contract, we both signed it and it stated that he had to come every 2 weeks and pay a visit and check on us all to see we were all right. But he didn't do that, it was months and months before we got to see him and all that time I had no money from the social and I was just fretting not knowing what to do.

From Jason's viewpoint, the social workers who had played a part in placing him in the residential assessment centre failed to provide him with the support he needed when he found himself parenting alone back in the community: 'I was dumped in the community and that was it. Make your own way, like, do your own thing. I didn't want massive support. I only needed a friendly ear to talk to, no more than that. I got my benefits through and then I had no more social workers, that was it, all done and dusted.'

BECOMING A SOCIAL WORKER

Kuldeep, Barbara, Ellen, Jan and Trish traced their interest in social work to early family experiences. Kuldeep came to live in England from India when she was very young and gained her knowledge of social work as a child, from the encounters of her family members and their friends with social services. As members of a minority ethnic community they viewed social workers positively as people who 'helped you out'. It was the older generation who, in her experience, turned to social workers to help them with housing and filling out forms. When they found they were unable to help themselves or use a welfare system they did not understand, not least because it was delivered linguistically and culturally in unfamiliar ways, social workers helped them.

Kuldeep went to college and trained as a nurse, a career she pursued for 10 years, working with older people. When she left to have her children she found herself becoming involved, as a mother, in local activities, running playgroups, starting nurseries and becoming a school governor.

The close-knit family and community she came from taught her that 'we had to do things for ourselves, no one else would do it for us'. Then her life 'came apart' and finding herself a lone parent, she needed to get back into paid work. She decided that social work might be a career in which the skills and knowledge she had developed as a mother would be useful. She went back to college and then onto a social work course, in the late 1990s, where she gained experience in a family centre and a residential unit working with children. These experiences confirmed to her that her future career lay in social work with families and children.

Barbara was the eldest daughter of a mother with disabilities. She recalls being bullied as a child because of her family's poverty. She learnt at an early age about what it was to be the carer of someone who faced oppression because of their disability and someone who needed help filling in forms to get financial help. Barbara married at 17 years of age and worked in the textile industry, winding yarn for 20 years as she brought up her four children. She describes herself as 'wanting better for her kids and pushing them into valuing education'. One of her daughters (while she was at college training to be a nursery nurse) arranged for Barbara to do an English language course. So at 39, Barbara started further education. After getting O levels, she was persuaded by a sociology tutor to take an access course in order to go to Nottingham Polytechnic. She took the plunge and left her job to become a mature student.

While getting her first degree Barbara decided she wanted to go further and enter social work training. This choice was informed by the fact that she had been a foster-mother for a nephew with learning disabilities: 'He did a lot for me and my family, my children grew up to be better people for the experience of helping someone less fortunate than them.' This experience had taught her to 'fight for his cause', getting him the services he needed to flourish, and through it she discovered that she wanted to do something about injustices and support vulnerable children. 'I'm not a do-gooder; it's about justice and what's right.' She did her social work training at Sheffield University and on qualification looked for a job with people who had learning disabilities. But when she didn't get one, she applied for a temporary post in a local children's team and then was asked if she wanted to work with disabled children. Three years later, when the services were reorganised, a specialist team for disabled children was created and Barbara found herself working across the range of children's work.

Ellen's mother was a home help and Ellen became a home care aide in her early teens: 'I would be doing little errands for people and helping her out really.' Her father was an active trade unionist and her experiences of the industrial action he was engaged in contributed to her emerging political awareness. Choosing social work, for Ellen, was about 'true socialist principles about helping people that are stuck in all sorts of difficult situations, in poverty, unemployment, and poor housing'. In the mid-1970s, she combined working in a children's home with going to college and then did a 4-year degree in social work. After working at Women's Aid for 3 years, she moved to work in a team that was setting up one of the earliest fostering schemes for 'troubled adolescents' and remembers feeling a sense of excitement and ownership about the service she was helping to create. She went on to work in the fostering team because of the flexibility it gave her as a parent:

> I have been able to have time out when I needed to. I have been able to work part-time when I want to, and I have also done little bits when I have acted up when we were a manager down and two of us shared that for a while. So there has been change within the work pattern for me. I have a sister who is quite dependent – she has a disability and she has a daughter who has Down's Syndrome so that has been quite a commitment there and then my own children have always been a lovely part of my life. So it has been a nice opportunity to combine a career along with a very deep-rooted sense of family.

Jan left school with little idea of what she wanted to do although she loved art. Her grandfather had a spell in a local psychiatric hospital and Jan applied for a job as a handicraft instructor at the hospital, which she thought would give her a chance to be creative and work directly with people. She moved from there into unqualified generic social work in 1974, with the encouragement of her colleagues. On her social work course, she had a placement working therapeutically with children which made her decide that her future was in child care social work.

Trish's interest in social work with children stemmed from her contact as the babysitter of a lad who was 'distressed and disturbed'. She felt she 'clicked with him' and when she was 18, she applied to work in a special school as a house-mother, moving on to an observational assessment centre at 20 and then into education qualifying her for social work. She considers that her interest in working with children and their families stemmed from the fact that 'I had a mum and dad who were the same all the way through my life. I didn't suffer any kind of abuse or real trauma, and I wanted to help people who didn't seem to have that kind of ordinary upbringing.'

Margaret, Sheila, Sue and Vicky thought about social work as a career because they developed interests in working with people through school and university. Margaret locates her decision to be a social worker in her Christian beliefs and the community-visiting she did when she was at school. Her headmistress tried to dissuade her from social work because it wasn't considered 'a good enough career ambition'. But she persisted and following a degree in social administration, she got a job in 1974 as an unqualified generic social worker and was seconded onto a qualifying social work course.

In her first degree in social sciences, one of Sheila's lecturers was a part-time social worker and because of this woman's stimulating teaching, Sheila decided to try social work for herself. She first worked with young people with learning disabilities and went on a qualifying social work course with the intention of staying in the learning disability field. But her placement experiences on the course made her change track and apply for a first qualified post in child care in 1989 in a child care team that worked 'across the range', from assessment through to adoption.

Vicky, like Sheila, came into social work because of the interest she developed in social sciences in her early 20s.

> I left school at 15. I was horse mad – all I ever wanted to do was work with horses. I tried to open up my own business, running a livery yard for horses, but that fell flat on its face. So I got a job in a pub, near a high-security prison, and a lot of prison officers used to come in and talk about the inmates. I found it quite fascinating and it made me think about doing psychology.

After getting psychology at A level, Vicky decided to go to university and do a social work course. When she completed it, she applied for a social work post working with children and families.

For Sue, an economics degree had led her to take up a job as a market researcher in an insurance company. But she did not feel fulfilled in this job compared with a friend from university who was working in child care social work. It was this friend's influence that led Sue in 1969 to apply for a trainee child care officer's job, and then a place on a social work course. Sue discovered after she had worked in social work for many years that her father had spent part of his childhood living with his siblings in a Dr Barnardo's village[3] where his widowed mother was a house-mother. Her father did not tell her about this until he was in his 80s and when he did she thought 'he was quite proud that I had become a social worker'.

SOCIAL WORKERS DESCRIBE THEIR WORK

The combined social work experience of the contributors spans the full range of children and family work across almost 4 decades. The accounts they gave of these experiences provided a rich source of data about the impact of policy, organisational and legal changes in social work with children and families.

Working with child sexual abuse

Jan and Margaret have been doing children and family work for over 30 years. Jan moved from working in neighbourhood-based generic teams to specialist child care posts including child protection. In the late 1980s, she was part of an initiative in her local authority to establish a specialist child sexual abuse social work team. It aimed to provide a resource of experienced, specialist social workers to work with this emerging area of concern for social services. It also provided support, consultation and training for mainstream child care social workers in issues relating to child sexual abuse. Despite subsequent reorganisations, Jan has been able to maintain this specialism and is currently the manager of a team of four social workers. She is enthusiastic about the work that she does:

> What gives me pleasure is that I'm the only manager with a case-load. I combine practice and management, supervising, teaching, everything, so it's unique really and because I have a practice case-load, I get paid less than everybody else! That's the punishment. I do direct work, consultation with people, training and service develop-ment. And that's just right for me. I am privileged to have a team of such calibre, I have excellent colleagues and we have students. I really enjoy case supervision and casework and training and teaching.

Jan describes her team as being 'shunted into a corner' compared to the high-profile areas in children and family work like adoption and fostering. But what detracts from her enjoyment with her job is the growth in the bureaucracy involved with children and family services as well as the endless policy and organisational changes that have emerged from the reforming agendas of recent governments. In her view, social work has learnt so much in relation to child protection work and risk, that what it needs now is stability, not change. It needs a chance to consolidate and build knowledge and confidence amongst its front-line practitioners. She feels that there is now a lack of recognition of the importance of social work values in local authority organisations. The current emphasis of managers on assessment work has been detrimental, in her judgement, to practitioners using their values, knowledge and skills to work long-term with families and make positive changes in their lives.

Margaret worked for 12 years as a generic social worker before a major reorganisation led her to choose working with children and families. She worked for a period as a child protection specialist providing support for mainstream child care social workers as well as working directly with children and families. A decade ago, she joined the specialist team that Jan manages. She works with children who have been sexually abused and with adults who have experienced abuse and are now parents. She also works at times with foster- and adoptive parents when a child's previous abuse becomes an issue. From her standpoint in a team that is connected to, but stands outside of, mainstream child protection and risk work, Margaret has concerns that working with the impact of child abuse has become a neglected area of social work. She is also worried that the organisation of services fragments the contacts between service users and social workers. In recent years, she has been increasingly aware of families who are passed from team to team and worker to worker, according to their status on the child protection register. In contrast to this, she says that her job satisfaction comes from

> . . . being able to do direct work with people and see change really, see both children and adults actually coming through it. It can be a very difficult process and the most successful cases I've had have been long-term, I mean over years. I have seen some of the adult women who have had hugely troubled pasts as children move on and start to live their lives and be able to parent the way they want or go on courses and do jobs when they have never been able to work before or get into better relationships. You can see change when you do this kind of work. Some of it involves enabling foster-carers and adopters to cope and manage. We may not always be working with the child directly but I really enjoy working with foster-carers and, increasingly, adoptive parents.

Working with crisis, risk and protection

Barbara, Kuldeep and Vicky all work at the front line of children and family social work: Barbara in a reception team, Kuldeep in a family support team, and Vicky in a community team where she is a senior practitioner. They work with a mix of other social workers and support workers, responding to family crises and carrying out risk assessments. Barbara describes it as 'fast-moving and pressured' work, not least because of staff vacancies in this area of children's work. There are lots of duty calls, which involve working with uncertainties and risks and having to make rapid assessments and judgements about possible options. She finds that she draws on her life experiences as well as her professional knowledge and training and it is a satisfying job for her:

> I love what I do. I am near to retiring age and I'll stay on until I'm 65. I never cease to marvel at the diverse range of people, who they are, what they do, what they say. I like the unexpected – you may have pre-formed opinions and you get out there and get the unexpected.

Kuldeep, like Barbara, gets 'a buzz' out of being in the front line of children and families' services. The work confirms her belief that people have the ability to change; that social workers can help people to achieve positive changes in their lives. She describes her work as making initial contacts and undertaking core assessments. She retains contact with people when child protection issues are identified; if not, she refers service users on to other teams. Kuldeep said that her work brings her into contact with many adults who lack the material, emotional and family resources to be the parents they would like to be. She recognises that services, as they are presently resourced and organised, cannot make up for these short-falls and this saddens her. Like many of the other social workers interviewed, she finds the expectations around paperwork make incredible inroads into her time and are repetitive. She said that the poor quality of the computer software that social workers are expected to use makes this aspect of the work 'very hard going'. She also identified a generation of managers in children and family work who do not have the depth and breadth of practice experience that their predecessors had as team managers. She feels that this means that new social workers as well as people like herself with 5 years or so of specialist experience are not getting the kind of in-depth supervision they need to develop their skills and confidence in the work they are doing.

Vicky also said that she finds the demands that have been made on her since she became a senior practitioner in a community children's team in 2004 'quite a ride'. She has to juggle with vacancies as well as a reorganisation that has taken place following the publication of *Every Child Matters* (Department for Education and Skills 2003). She anticipates that 'it's going to be chaos for a while' and said she wonders how the services are going to manage these changes.

Working in fostering and adoption

Whilst Sheila and Trish work in fostering teams, their routes into their posts included a number of years in the front line of children and families' work. Sheila began work as a qualified social worker in a generic child care team in 1989. Following a reorganisation of the children and families' services, she chose to work with 'looked-after' children.[4] After the birth of her third child, she decided to apply for a job-share so that she could work part-time, but before this could be organised, she went off sick with stress, as she outlines:

> I was at work one day and I suddenly felt sick and sweating. I felt panicky and I put down the phone on a birth parent who was swearing at me and threatening me and I said to my manager, 'I can't do this, I'm going home.'

Sheila had loved her job and was very committed to the children with whom she was working. But she felt that her job was having such a detrimental effect on her life that she had to do something about it. She subsequently returned to work in a more rural area where she hoped there might be less pressure. However, she found that, as one of the most experienced workers on the team, she was given a large caseload and she went off sick again. Three years ago, Sheila took a job in another Midlands local authority in a fostering team and found:

> ... it was the best decision I took, because it meant I got my health back, I got my family life back and I am still in social work, but doing a very different job. But all the skills I had from my child care experience are relevant to what I do now.

Sheila supervises social workers, assesses and trains foster-parents, and supports foster-parents who are experiencing difficulties. She is very positive about her job and her work environment and is impressed by the people who are applying to be foster-parents. She feels well supported but she continues to be concerned about what is happening in child protection services. She sees these services as

> ... allowing staff like myself, to be destroyed by the job. They need to look after people better. We are so short in the country of experienced child care workers. Services are increasingly staffed by very inexperienced, unqualified agency staff. It's all back-to-front. I often think, 'Why doesn't someone up top look down and think, Why is the fostering team full of all these really experienced people while the staff in the protection services are going off sick and there are vacancies?'

A reorganisation in the early 1990s faced Trish with a choice of working with either the under-8s or over-8s, a division which she and her colleagues struggled to make sense of. She chose the under-8s because she wanted to continue to do preventive work with children and families. But she found that most of the work that she was doing was child protection work and she became frustrated: 'I was always thinking – not enough time, not enough resources. The job was grinding me down.' After 8 years of this, she went off sick and later applied for a job in a fostering team. She has now held this job for 5 years and still finds the job fulfilling. She has the time to plan her work and build sustained relationships with the foster-families with whom she works. She has recently taken on a half-time management role in relation to the team's duty system and she spends the rest of the week supporting foster-families, maintaining placements and developing the service.

Ellen and Sue have both worked in fostering since the 1980s. They moved into fostering because, at that time, it was the only part of the local authority social services department that was offering part-time work to women with children. Ellen has covered most areas of fostering and adoption during her career. Her main role in the fostering team is working with a specialist scheme which arranges long-term fostering for children with disabilities. She also works in other areas, helping younger children who are moving on to adoption and assessing and training foster-parents for long-term placements. Ellen likes the variety of tasks she is asked to take on, and enjoys working in collaboration with health colleagues to enable children with disabilities to be looked after in the community. She also appreciates the support she gets from managers and colleagues:

> I think we are a real team. Many of us have been around a long time and there are a lot of part-time staff, so it is big. There are always people about and always someone to bounce ideas off and that I think is crucial.

Ellen finds there is less time for social workers to work directly with foster-parents than there used to be and there are fewer foster-carers to choose from when placements are made. The bureaucracy and form-filling have grown enormously:

> Our group manager has tried to reduce it, where she can, but every-thing has to be signed in triplicate and everything needs three forms before you can get it. When you are rushed with an assessment and you know that carer won't get paid unless you have done the form-filling, you do it to get the carer paid and your planning for that visit might be done in the car on the way to the visit. I am someone who likes to plan things so I do find it frustrating.

Sheila works in the same team as Ellen. When she was 60, she cut her time to 21 hours a week. She now supports foster-care staff, arranges emergency foster-placements and sits on adoption panels. She enjoys her work and feels well supported by her managers and colleagues. She finds social work more structured than it was in the past, and appreciates this: 'There is much more emphasis on forms and filling things in and doing things to a set pattern. Before, we did things a lot more by trial and error.' In her years with the same local authority, she has, like many of the other social workers interviewed for this chapter, gone through a series of re-organisations. She has seen offices move from being open and based in local communities to being located in places where they are cut off from local transport routes and protected from the public by window bars and security devices. She thinks that this means there are lost opportunities to interest local people in fostering and adoption.

LESSONS FOR THE FUTURE

The contributors to this chapter talked a great deal about the impact of scarce resources, problems of staff retention and recruitment and unending reorganisations of services on children and families in need. Yet despite the difficulties and traumas that result from this, all were clear that social work with children and families is an essential service requiring committed and knowledgeable workers, with the time and support to do the job for which they have been trained.

Jason said that social work is 'not the sort of job you do for the money. You've got to want to do a job like that, it's a serious job, and there are people with serious issues out there that need help, they need you to be there for them.' For David, what is important is that social workers 'find a way in their job to have the space and listen to the stories that people are struggling to tell them. If you allow yourself to get overloaded and you're running on empty, then you're no good to anyone.' The social workers in this chapter would agree. However, Trish and Sheila, who shared their personal experiences of overload and stress, argued strongly that dealing with the pressures of front line children and families' work was not solely a matter for individual practitioners. They argued that trans-formation is needed in the resourcing, the organisation and, above all, the management and supervision of practitioners. As Sheila commented:

> We are not going to retain people and recruit high-calibre people in social work if we don't recognise what they do, look after them, value them, support them, and make them feel that what they do is a good job.

The social workers were hopeful that the integration of social work with health and education services will be good news for children and families. Jan added that other issues need to be taken on board:

> For the future, I think, we need to hold onto our social work values and the core of our knowledge and skills. But the climate around social work has to change to enable it to flourish. I would like to see people who are in the profession and in training trying to create a climate where people can flourish at this work, rather than struggle. There will never be enough money for social work, but we can create the conditions where we can enable workers to feel strong, positive, confident, able to be good advocates, able to do the work, enjoy it

and promote it. I think with the integration agenda now we have opportunities to stand up and be strong, but we need people to be able to promote the profession within a group where health and education will be dominant. So we've got a challenge ahead because social work has been a very quiet profession generally and I think it's time we changed that.

ACKNOWLEDGEMENTS

Our thanks go to Janice Foulds, Bert Pollheimer, Lynda Stone and Heather Livesey for taking the time to arrange interviews with social workers and Linda Ward for making connections for us with service users.

NOTES

1 Children's Guardians are qualified social workers who are experienced in working with children and families in England and Wales. They are appointed by the court to represent the rights and interests of children in cases that involve social services. See http://www.cafcass.gov.uk/.
2 Under section 17 of the Children Act 1989, local authorities have a general duty to safeguard and protect the welfare of children and promote the upbringing of children by their families, by providing a range and level of services appropriate to those children's needs. This can include making direct payments or providing vouchers if social workers are able to make a case for such provision.
3 Barnardo's village in Berkshire provided homes to needy children between 1878 and 1986. See http://www.goldonian.org/barkingside/tvh_1930_40.htm
4 This term applies to all children who are supervised by a council when they are subject to a supervision requirement, order, authorisation or warrant under the provisions of the Children Act 1989 and the Children (Scotland) Act 1995, or they are being provided with accommodation under the same Acts.

REFERENCES

Butler, I. and Drakeford, M. (2005) *Scandal, Social Policy and Social Welfare*, 2nd edition, Bristol: Policy Press/British Association of Social Workers.
Davis, A. and Wainwright, S. (2005) 'Combating Poverty and Social Exclusion: Implications for Social Work Education', *Social Work Education*, 24(3): 259–73.
Department for Education and Skills (2003) *Every Child Matters*, Cm. 5860, London: the Stationery Office.
Department of Health and Department for Education and Skills (2004) *National Service Framework for Children, Young People and Maternity Services*, London: the Stationery Office.
Featherstone, B. (2004) *Family Life and Family Support: A Feminist Analysis*, Basingstoke: Palgrave Macmillan.

Garrett, P. (2003) *Remaking Social Work with Children and Families: A Critical Discussion on the Modernisation of Social Care*, London: Routledge.

Joseph Rowntree Foundation (December 2005) *Monitoring Poverty and Social Exclusion in the UK*, York: JRF.

Laming, Lord (January 2003) *The Victoria Climbié Inquiry: Report of an Inquiry*, Secretary of State for Health and the Secretary of State for the Home Department, London: the Stationery Office.

Morris, K. (2005) 'From "Children in Need" to "Children at Risk". The Changing Policy Context for Prevention and Participation', *Practice*, 17(2): 70–6.

Preston, G. (ed.) (2005) *At Greatest Risk: the Children Most Likely to be Poor*, London: Child Poverty Action Group.

Secretary of State for Health (2003) *Keeping Children Safe: the Government's Response to the Victoria Climbié Report and the Joint Chief Inspectors' Report, 'Safeguarding Children'*, Cm. 5861, London: the Stationery Office.

Sinclair, I. (2005) *Fostering Now: Messages from Research*, London: Jessica Kingsley Publishing.

Chapter 3

Criminal justice social work

INTRODUCTION

This chapter presents an aspect of social work practice which exists within Scotland, but which is organised very differently in other parts of the UK. In Scotland, offender services are social work services, unlike the rest of the UK. Moore and Whyte (1998) argue that the organisation, delivery and philosophy behind social work in Scotland are unique within the UK and within the world. They suggest that the reason for this lies in the Social Work (Scotland) Act of 1968 which determined that responsibilities for 'probation type' services would lie with agencies which 'had a duty, first and foremost, to promote well-being within the community' (1998: 15). In consequence, work with offenders was established as a social work service, carried out by qualified social workers, within the context of mainstream social work services.

This is not to suggest that this arrangement is fixed and for all time. A review of criminal justice social work was held in 2004–5, leading to the passing of the Management of Offenders (Scotland) Act 2005. This Act created eight criminal justice authorities from 1 April 2006, and a National Advisory Board, chaired by the Justice Minister. The legislation requires that criminal justice social work and the prison service should work together in the future, but is not a merger of prison and probation services as institutionalised in England and Wales in the establishment of the National Offender Management Service (NOMS).[1]

The fact that offender services are social work services should not lead the reader to assume that Scotland is 'soft on crime'. Scotland's prison figures indicate that in 2004–5, the average daily population in Scottish prisons totalled 6,779, the highest annual level ever recorded. Over the 9-year period from 1996–7 to 2004–5, the average daily prison population increased by 13 per cent. In the same 9-year period, the female prison population increased by 75 per cent; over six times the growth which was experienced in the male prison population (Scottish

Executive 2005). Scotland's prison population reached its highest recorded level of 7,072 in March 2004 (news report in *The Scotsman*, 25 November 2005).

What we have, then, is a set of rather mixed messages in Scotland about crime, punishment and welfare. The consequence for those working in the criminal justice services is that they can feel torn, at times, between conflicting ideologies, as our contributors demonstrate. Nevertheless, the contributors are, on the whole, proud of the achievements of criminal justice social work. They welcome the existence of the National Objectives and Standards[2] which provide the framework for service delivery, and while the pace of change in the criminal justice social work service over the last 10 years has been described as 'striking' (Moore and Whyte 1998), change has been underpinned by an attempt to do things better; to create a service which is based on evidence of 'what works' in criminal justice. This has been demonstrated by the introduction of programmes based on cognitive behavioural principles for medium-risk and high-risk offenders (see Burnett and Roberts 2004, Raynor 2004) as well as the development of new diversion programmes; programmes which are designed to keep offenders out of prison and in the community. Restorative justice schemes (see McLaughlin *et al.* 2003) and Drug Treatment and Testing Orders (see Hough *et al.* 2003, Windlesham 2001) are two such initiatives which will be discussed in this chapter.

THE CONTRIBUTORS

All the contributors to this chapter live in Scotland, and most live in and around Edinburgh. In their individual stories, they illustrate specific aspects of the working of criminal justice social work services in Scotland. They also, however, offer comment on probation as it is delivered throughout the UK, and indeed, make a contribution to general debates about the role of criminal justice in society.

Service users

Donna

I'm 24, I've got two kids, one in primary school and one just coming up to nursery, and in the future, I hope to start college, to become a legal secretary – that's what I'd like to do. I've got a probation officer and a children and families' social worker right now.

Mark

I live in Edinburgh and I'm 29 years old and a spray painter for a well-recognised company in Edinburgh. I'm single, no children, have my own flat, lost my driving licence, have a girlfriend. I'm currently on probation for 2 years and have a 5-year ban from driving.

Neil

I live in Musselburgh, outside Edinburgh, and work night-shift as a community psychiatric nurse in a local psychiatric hospital. My story goes back to 4 years ago when I was violently attacked by a group of teenage girls. I took part in mediation after this.

Practitioners

Alison

I'm 30, I'm from Fife. I grew up in a medium-sized town but wanted to move to a bigger city, so moved to Edinburgh. I started working in criminal justice social work just 6 months ago, and now work part-time in the main office and half a week seconded to the group work programme.

Arlon

I am a social worker with 30 years' experience, have always practised in Scotland, apart from a brief time in Northern Ireland. I am currently a team leader in criminal justice social work services in Fife. I am also a mother of three and a part-time PhD student. I like to play music – I play classical guitar, just for fun.

Fiona

I live in Edinburgh and work as a senior social worker for the Drug Treatment and Testing Order programme. I enjoy life. I am doing the post-graduate MSc in Criminal Justice at the University of Edinburgh; I've just finished the second year of this.

Hector

I am 40 years old, started studying for social work only 5 years ago, and have been qualified now for approaching 3 years. I've been in criminal justice all that time. I spend 2 days a week running probation groups from a central office and the rest of the time at my own office providing a service to the court and managing licences.

Niall

I work and live in Edinburgh. I work for a non-governmental organisation, SACRO,[3] in the area of victim/offender mediation. I am white, educated, middle-class, Irish (from the South of Ireland). I lived in Northern Ireland for many years.

Ron

I have been involved in social work for 34 years in Scotland. I like to do the best I can personally in my endeavours in my profession and personal life. I am currently manager of criminal justice social work services for the City of Edinburgh council.

Sarah

I've worked in criminal justice since I qualified in 1996. I've always worked in Edinburgh, and I now manage the probation group work programme. I'm 33. I was born and brought up in Edinburgh, but now live outside the city.

EXPERIENCING CRIME

Service users in criminal justice social work come from two very different groups. They are either those who commit crimes (often called offenders or perpetrators of crime) or they are those who suffer the effects of crime, known as crime victims. This separation is, at some times and in some places, rather an artificial one. Critical sociologists have pointed out that much routine criminal justice is focused on the behaviour of young, poor, working-class people, who are predominantly male, and who may experience crime as both victims and offenders (Cree 2000, Maguire *et al.* 2002). Likewise, recent research suggests that those who commit violent crime are likely to have had personal experience of violence against them in the past (Smith 2004).

This is not in any way to minimise the devastating impact of crime. As the stories in this chapter demonstrate, being a victim of crime brings shock and devastation to people's lives, and may require a major reassessment of priorities and lifestyle. When Neil was assaulted, the attack came out of the blue. He explains:

> My story goes back to 4 years ago when I was visiting a friend, it was a Saturday night, on my way home, I was violently attacked by a group of teenage girls. It was a completely unprovoked attack, they gave me a good beating, which lasted about 15 minutes, I was

hospitalised and off work for 7 months. Although the physical injuries disappeared quite quickly, I was left with quite deep-seated psychological issues.

The assault made Neil afraid to leave his house, and his confidence was shattered, not least because the attack had come from a group of girls, two of whom were under 16 years of age.

Mark's experience was very different to this. Crime was, for him, less of an isolated, unexpected event, and more a way of life as he was growing up. It is only recently that he has begun to see his past behaviour as problematic. He puts it as follows:

> I've been a bit up and down in the past, and repeated a lot of mistakes. I'm not a stupid person, I've got intelligence, but I've never learned from my mistakes in the past, that's been my downfall. A lot of it has been fun, but it has also caused me a lot of upheaval. I could have done better in life, got further in life, if I hadn't gone the road I did, getting involved in recreational drugs when I was younger. I've never been a smack user, I've always been a worker, apart from a few glitches – I believe you've got to work, to be the same as everybody else out there – even when work is boring – it makes the world go round.

Mark's account illustrates some features which are frequently present in the lives of young offenders. We can clearly see his strengths – his ability to hold down a job, his engaging personality and his personal insight. We can also see that for Mark, involvement in crime (that is, recreational drugs) was part of normal behaviour, not seen as noteworthy or necessarily 'criminal', except that he now realises that it had held him back in life.

Donna also has a long history of involvement in crime and criminal justice. She explained that she developed an addiction to heroin following her mother's death, and shoplifted to get money to feed her addiction:

> I was 21 when my mum passed away, she had cancer, and because of all the stress, I ended up taking heroin, and shoplifting – I was shoplifting nearly every day, and I kept getting arrested by the police. I was put up in front of the sheriff as much as three times a week – kept getting bailed to appear at a later date, and then I would never appear. The courts were really busy at the time. I started at the District Court then moved up to the Sheriff Court and eventually I was remanded for not appearing in court, and that was when a social worker first got involved with me – I spent five weeks in Cornton Vale prison.

HM Institution Cornton Vale is Scotland's only female prison. It reached notoriety in 1997 when the seventh suicide in 30 months was reported; this was at a time when the prison population was 170 remand and convicted prisoners. This shocking statistic led to a review (Social Work Services and Prisons Inspectorate for Scotland 1998) which called for alternative, community-based measures for women offenders. By the time of the annual inspection of the prison in 2005, the prison population had risen to 340. The Chief Inspector of Prisons in Scotland, Dr Andrew McLellan, declared: 'Cornton Vale holds very many prisoners with a high incidence of drug addiction (estimated 98 per cent), mental health problems (estimated 80 per cent), history of abuse (estimated 75 per cent) and very poor physical health.' He went on to ask: 'What will prison do for them?'[4] This question is an important one for us to consider when we look at what service users have found helpful.

WHAT HELPS?

Perhaps more than in any other field of social work practice, the users of criminal justice services are likely, in the words of Trotter (1999), to be 'involuntary clients': they do not ask to receive services; instead, services are imposed on them by a court order or threat of some other legal action.

Probation services

Mark first came to the attention of the police when he was 15 years of age, pushing a motorbike through a small town in the Borders of Scotland. He denied driving the motorbike, but a hot engine told otherwise, and he was subsequently charged with having no insurance and no licence, and was banned from driving. Over the next 14 years, although he managed to remain in employment for most of the time, Mark received a further three driving bans, and spent time in prison as a result of a drug offence. At the time of interview, Mark had been on probation for 18 months and, during this time, he had met a criminal justice social worker on a regular basis (monthly at first and then bi-monthly). He had also attended two intensive probation groups, one on alcohol and the other on car crime. He feels that it is only now that he has received the help that he needed all along:

> I think it was good for me personally being put into the social work system, to the two groups, the way it's worked out, because that's changed my whole perspective and attitude to my life, but I do feel a wee bit let down that if this had happened to me when I was 21 and I was getting in trouble and gathering up my criminal record,

maybe if I had been put into this before now, I maybe wouldn't have been involved in the stuff I have been involved in.

Mark believes that the individual support provided by the criminal justice social worker and the intensive experience of the groups were of critical importance in helping him to confront his attitudes and life-style and begin to make changes in the way that he behaves. He explains first how important his relationship is with Pam, his criminal justice social worker:

> If I got in trouble now, I'd feel that I'd let Pam down – like your mum and your dad – that's the kind of relationship that it is. I'd be disappointed that I'd disappointed her.

He then describes the alcohol group, run by voluntary agency SACRO:

> I listened, and participated, and contributed – and the more you put in, the more you enjoy it and the more you get out of it as well. It was really beneficial for me. It wasn't, 'Don't drink' – it was educating you, telling you all the dangers and the 'bads' and 'goods' about drinking – they were pointing out the health factors, how to control alcohol use – so, 'If you're going to drink, watch how you drink, and be careful', which was good. They were just trying to get you to do it the right way and the sensible way, not telling you not to do it. If you go over the score, you end up spoiling it or getting into bother – when someone has had too much to drink, the chances are that there will be some kind of negativity, whether you're getting upset, or falling and hurting yourself, or something like that.

Mark benefited from the whole package available to him, what has been called a 'multi-modal' approach (see Burnett and Roberts 2004). The one-to-one relationship with the social worker was central in allowing him to explore feelings about himself, his partner, his family and his life. After some years out of favour, criminal justice social work has recently rehabilitated the idea of the importance of relationship (see Perlman 1979), often described in the language of 'pro-social modelling' (Trotter 1999). A criminal justice social worker, Hector, outlines what pro-social modelling means to him in his work:

> You've got to use yourself, but you've also got to be very careful that you're not just venting stories of your own life that don't have any purpose. I feel comfortable enough with the things that I can and do share – but you can do so without identifying yourself within

those experiences. You've got to be prepared to say, 'Yeh, I did this, or I did that, I thought this', because you are asking people to share with you, so you've got to be prepared to share with them as well.

Mark also enjoyed the group work, which is an aspect of criminal justice social work which has flourished over the last 10 years or so. Group work programmes which use learning theory and cognitive psychology, and focus on faulty thinking and reasoning, and teach problem-solving skills, have been championed as more effective than conventional approaches to reducing reoffending (see Roberts 2004). Whether or not this is the case (and there is a live debate about this), such programmes have proliferated in prison and probation settings. The manager of probation group work programmes in Edinburgh, Sarah, demonstrates that group work's success is not only about cognitive reasoning; it is also about relationships and support:

> I can think of one guy – he was lovely, but it was *awful* the things that he'd done. He attempted to murder someone . . . He had such a horrible history. Both parents had died of AIDS before he was 12, he was brought up by a series of aunts and grannies and, like so many of the guys we work with, he'd been in residential care, ended up in Polmont[5] really early, and then went in and out of jail. None of us thought that he'd have managed the group – he had a terrible life – his girlfriend had had a baby, and then she was killed in a car crash. He stabbed someone, they stabbed him, he was forever showing his wounds. At the time, he was a drug user (on heroin, I think) and living in homeless accommodation, and yet he got here every single day – it was a space for him to come. He was really good at art – he drew pictures for us at break times and we encouraged all that. He completed the programme, and has never come back – he seems to have moved on. Having the consistent support here made a difference.

Straight talking

Donna's story provides another aspect of what helps in social work. She tells the story of the police breaking down her front door one night, accusing her partner of dealing in drugs. When they found that there were children in the house, they contacted the children and families' social work team. A case conference was held soon afterwards, and the children were placed on the 'at risk' child protection register. Donna relates the conversation with the social worker:

> I said I was really worried about losing the kids and she says to me, 'The only way you will lose them, will be by your actions – it's totally up to you. I know that you can't change your life overnight, but we will help you.'

Donna welcomed her social worker's 'straight talking', and was pleased that she had placed responsibility firmly with her. Donna was also appreciative of the fact that the social worker lived up to her promise of giving help. She continues:

> And they *have* helped me. My daughter goes to a group now on a Thursday – it's a group for children whose parents are on methadone prescriptions – they can talk to each other about what's going on, or they can just play. She really loves it. They pick her up from school in a taxi and they drop her off here at 6 p.m. in a taxi. I got a letter this morning for my son to go to nursery – he is young for starting nursery, but it's a social work nursery and everyone says it'll be great for him.

The 'down-side' for Donna is the number of professionals now involved in her life. She has five different 'social work' personnel coming to her flat: a children and families' social worker, a criminal justice social worker, a drugs counsellor, a health visitor and her partner's Drug Treatment and Testing Order worker. This can be 'overwhelming' for her:

> At times, I've been a bit overwhelmed with all the appointments, and at times, especially when it concerns children and families, I feel as if I've just got a big rucksack on my back full of bricks, because I'm constantly worried about what's going to happen with the kids.

Mediation services

As a victim of a serious assault, Neil elected to take part in a process of mediation, in which he met face-to-face with the young women who had badly injured him. The sheriff made mediation a condition of the sentence on the four young women, thus making criminal history in Scotland. SACRO was allocated the case, and a social worker acted as intermediary between Neil and his assailants, preparing all parties for meeting each other, and debriefing them afterwards. Neil explains what was helpful about his SACRO social worker:

> It was his humanity, his warmth and his acceptance. He has such empathy – he's very easy to relate to and to talk to. He just took me

at my level, allowed me to take my time, if I got upset that was OK, it was all at my pace, and I appreciated that. I didn't feel pressured, he just went with me every step of the way – I felt he was a good support. It was important to me that I didn't hold back – but you need to have the trust to be able to do that.

Neil was acutely aware that the social worker was also using his interpersonal skills with his assailants, but his belief in the social worker's professionalism was strong enough for him not to worry unduly about this:

He had to build the same relationship with the girls – so that they would trust him. I knew they met, but not what they spoke about, but I knew that whatever they did, they did for a purpose, that it was for the common good – I had confidence in him.

Neil eventually had two meetings with his attackers, two of the young women attending the first meeting and the other two the second, accompanied by their mothers. Neil outlines what happened:

The meetings were quite informal. I came into the room, the girls were already there waiting for me, we all sat in a circle, we introduced ourselves, said who we were, the girls had the opportunity to speak first, from their point of view, what happened, then I gave them my story, told them how I felt and how it had affected me, and the social worker summed up and off we went. It took about 45 minutes to an hour. It was very open; once I started talking, I couldn't stop. I was very calm and controlled – I wasn't upset or nervous – it was like throwing a switch and all this came out.

Neil understands what made these meetings a success. His friends had urged him not to go ahead; they were afraid that he might be hurt all over again. Even his social worker had advised him that things could go one of two ways: either there would be a good dialogue, or the young women might say nothing. But, as Neil narrates, 'It didn't happen that way though, because the social worker had prepared the girls well.' It was the care and, above all, the preparation which had made this process a positive one, not just for Neil, but for the young women who had attacked him. They expressed considerable remorse at the meetings, as did their mothers. (Neil said he saw the mothers as victims themselves.) Neil has gone on to become a volunteer for SACRO, meeting other victims and offenders and talking about his experiences at national conferences on restorative justice.

BECOMING A SOCIAL WORKER

Some of the criminal justice social workers whom we met, in common with contributors in other chapters, cite the influence of family and upbringing as significant in their subsequent career choice. Fiona's mother worked with older people, and helped her to find work in social care settings before she went to university and during the holidays. Although she studied Business Management at university, Fiona subsequently worked in residential settings with adults with learning disabilities, and found herself gravitating towards social work as a career. Arlon grew up in Glasgow in what she describes as 'a very Red Clyde-side Labour-orientated family, which had a trade union aspect to it. My grandfather was one of the first to join the Dockers' Union in Glasgow.' Arlon went to university to study Philosophy, Sociology and Psychology, and during this time, encouraged by her mother, she worked for a summer as a volunteer community worker in Belfast. It was this experience which cemented her decision to become a social worker.

Two contributors said that they had not thought about a career in social work until it was suggested to them by a careers' officer. So, a careers' master at Ron's school had shown him a leaflet about social work. This was in the late 1960s and, as he said, 'an exciting time, with the introduction of the Social Work (Scotland) Act and the creation of new social work departments'. He continues:

> I didn't know any social workers at that time. But I knew that I didn't want to work behind a bank counter. I can't say there was a blinding inspiration, because there wasn't. Before that time, I'd heard of probation, and knew about the man from 'the Cruelty',[6] or the woman from 'the Welfare',[7] but this was all changing with the new Act. My parents were both involved in the church. But I was a bit more of a rebel at that time – I was into guitars and rock and roll.

Alison came into social work 30 years later. When she left school, she wasn't sure what she wanted to do, except that she hoped for 'a job where I wasn't doing the same thing every day', because she had found school boring – 'not the subjects, as much as the structure'. A careers' officer gave her a leaflet on social work, but she did not act on it at this time, and instead, went off to India as a volunteer to work on a rural technology project, 'building mud ovens, learning about water conservation, that kind of thing'. When she came back to Scotland, she worked in various unqualified social care jobs, until she embarked on her training at 24 years of age.

Some social workers spent considerable amounts of time in alternative careers, before entering social work. Hector did not begin social work until he was 35 years of age. He had grown up in South Africa, and had worked in the construction industry for many years, also spending some years as a professional footballer. He drifted into social work with, as he says, 'no particular intentions':

> I moved over to the UK, I hadn't liked what I'd been doing for a number of years, was not stimulated by it, and thought, 'What can I do?' When I got to the UK, there were a lot of small colleges offering courses. I was working as a barman, staying with a friend, thought I needed to do something that would sustain me – I suppose I was thinking, 'This is my last chance now, I'm getting on a bit, I need to make a final decision.' So I looked at computer courses, saw Open University stuff, and the material on social work interested me – the course was called 'Health and Social Care'. I knew nothing about it, or where it might take me, or what the qualification was at the end of this. I didn't even know what social workers did!

Niall's journey into social work was more deliberate, and yet perhaps just as fundamental a life-change. He had joined the Catholic priesthood at 18 years of age, and trained and worked in Ireland and Northern Ireland for many years before coming to Edinburgh 8 years ago to begin social work training. His decision to leave the priesthood and become a social worker was a gradual one. Early in his work as a priest, he referred a child who had been abused to the social work department, and was impressed by the personal qualities and professionalism of the social worker who had dealt with the case. But his decision to change direction was brought to a head by 'a terrible shooting which took place in a little village where I used to live'. In 1994, six Catholics were gunned down as they sat in O'Toole's public house in Loughinisland, County Down, to watch the World Cup. Niall takes up the story:

> The repercussions were huge. I realised then that whatever I could offer as a priest, it wasn't enough for me, so I actively began to train in a skilled way to care for people in distress and need. I trained as a counsellor in Belfast for 3 years, and I practised as a counsellor in North Belfast. I helped to set up – I was one of the first team of counsellors at – a voluntary service in Ardoyne, another area full of distress. I subsequently decided to move full-time into social work and came to Edinburgh to train.

Sarah's account demonstrates that different kinds of social work attract different kinds of people. She explains:

I've never really wanted to be a social worker – I wanted to work with offenders – I don't know why! I never had any deep realisation that I wanted to help people, then when I was at university we had a chance to go into Castle Huntly Prison[8] as a support thing for the prisoners, and I really, really liked it – I liked the interaction with folk. There was a group and you talked and did activities with them, once a month, I went along with my friend, out of curiosity as much as anything – getting inside a jail. I did that for a year. From that, I decided I'd like to work with offenders, and in Scotland, there's no probation service, so it was criminal justice social work. I suppose what I really wanted was to be a probation officer.

SOCIAL WORKERS DESCRIBE THEIR WORK

Ron sets the scene for criminal justice social work services in Edinburgh:

Our service is about undertaking a range of assessments for courts and parole boards and for any other requirement of assessment on people who are offending; to assist courts and other decision-making bodies to arrive at the best outcome in that case, or the most appropriate outcome in that case. In other words, the 3,500 reports that we do here in Edinburgh are to assist, by law, the sentencers; to help them determine the most appropriate sentence. That's what they're doing. They're also pointing out levels of risk, risk of reoffending, risk of custody . . .

On the intervention side, it's twofold. We have the community service intervention side – the alternative to imprisonment – the reparation stuff – there's a penalty on offenders' time and they go and 'do good' in the community to pay off what they have done wrong. So in Edinburgh, we have 1,000 men and women on community service at any one given time, and they are going around doing their work. That's tangible because you can see it, you can measure it. . . . What happens on probation? On a one-to-one probation order, I think that's a very good question – what does happen on probation? Because if you are involved in a short action plan, I would argue strongly that some people require an intervention that is *welfare* orientated. To deny that is discriminatory. I don't think that's old social work hat – tosh! – it's what that person may require. Running alongside that now, we have things called group work and intensive intervention programmes running for under-21s, and for over-21s – these programmes are based on cognitive intervention methodology.

In this outline, Ron touches on a number of themes which are developed in the accounts of the social workers. We will begin with assessment and, more specifically, assessment of risk.

Assessment/risk assessment

Fiona worked at Glenochil Prison[9] before moving to manage the Drug Treatment and Testing Order (DTTO) service for Edinburgh. All those with whom she worked in prison had been convicted of serious offences and were on long sentences of 4 years or more. A key part of her role was assessing the men's readiness for parole. Under the terms of the Prisoners and Criminal Proceedings (Scotland) Act 1993, prisoners sentenced to 4 years or more are eligible to be considered for release on parole once they have served half their sentence. Those who are not freed on parole are usually released once they have served two-thirds of their sentence.[10] Fiona said that she worried 'all the time' about public safety, and did not recommend parole very often. But prisoners were then released on 'non-parole licence', and this raised inevitable safety issues.

In her current job, Fiona is again assessing offenders, but this time assessment is in the context of their drug use. DTTOs were first introduced to Scotland in 1999 (October 2000 in the rest of the UK) as a high tariff disposal for drug-misusing offenders who might otherwise receive a custodial sentence.[11] The intention was to tackle those whose offending is a direct result of their drug-misuse, that is, those who steal to fund their habit. DTTOs have two objectives: to reduce crime and to reduce drug misuse, as Fiona outlines:

> The idea is that we get people in on court orders who are using heroin to excess, offending to excess and whose lives are completely and utterly chaotic. We try to stabilise all that, by offering an intensive service. People attend at least four times a week in the early stages, and go to court every month, to see if the order continues.

The DTTO project is multi-disciplinary; social workers supervise offenders and deal with all the statutory and legal requirements. As Fiona wryly states: 'We're the big bad wolves, because if anything goes wrong, we have to tell people.' When the project began, many of those whose orders were breached by social workers ended up back in prison. That is less likely today, with sheriffs preferring to try different community disposals, such as community service or a fine. Fiona is realistic about what progress is for those with whom she is working:

> We're making huge progress with some of our clients – even if it's going from injecting to smoking heroin, that's a huge positive.

Success in criminal justice social work?

Hector works half-time in probation group work and half-time in regular criminal justice social work activities. Asked about effectiveness, he talked passionately:

> I think we should stand up and say jail doesn't work – it leads people to become more hardened offenders, 100 times over . . . Social work needs to influence the debate at ministerial level; to tell the public, 'This is what changes behaviour, this is what reduces offending, give us time and then maybe we can prove that to you.' And then the courts should be given the latitude to make those kinds of decisions. At the moment, courts are pressurised to be hard, and I think we need to become more vocal and central to the debate about offending.

Alison had only been qualified for 6 months at the point where she was interviewed for the book. She said that it is difficult to pinpoint success in criminal justice social work:

> In community care, if you find a good nursing home for someone, it's tangible. Within criminal justice, you cannot view success just on whether someone reoffends or not, because the majority of our clients are reoffending all the time, they've got a lot of drug abuse, lots of situations where they are choosing to reoffend all the time. My personal view as a newly qualified worker is that success is where someone's attitudes have changed, their motivations have increased, they are able to identify where they want to *be* – for a lot of our clients, they are going through the same routines, the same motions day after day, week after week, year after year, and they have no thoughts – because there is so much crisis going on in their lives all the time, they have never had time out to stop and think, 'Where am I aiming to be? What am I trying to do? What's the point of my existence?' When people haven't got something to aim for and a challenge and something they're trying to achieve, they've not got the motivation to try and live an offence-free life . . . If we can motivate people to want something out of their own life, and to feel that they can do something – that their destiny isn't defined for them – then I think we can make a big difference.

Alison believes that offence-focused work is fundamental to her practice, but that offence-focused work, to be effective, 'relies on people being open and honest not just with themselves but with you as well'. And to get that relationship, 'you have to build it'. She describes working with a man who was on probation for assaulting his mother:

... when he first came on probation, he was very resistant ... He was very reluctant to talk to me for a very long time, and would sit with his legs and his arms crossed and not say very much. As the weeks and months progressed, he began to talk and share a little bit more, to the point where, when it was time to reduce his contact to monthly, he said at the review, 'I don't want it reduced to monthly, I want it fortnightly because I have never spoken to anybody as honestly as I do here.' That was a big thing for me – I was quite taken aback, because it didn't seem a lot he was sharing with me, compared with other people.

The motivation to change

Although Arlon is now a manager of probation services, she has always stayed close to practice, because, as she said, she likes 'the nitty-gritty of the practical work'. In describing criminal justice social work, Arlon argues that people have to *want* to change; no amount of services will help someone unless they are ready to embrace change.[12] She describes a recent example of a young offender in Fife:

A young woman of 19 or 20 had been causing havoc – she had smashed all the plate glass windows in an office, had committed a serious assault with a knife against another woman, was completely out of control. We put in a whole load of packages of help, including sending her to a residential unit for a time. ... The change in her attitude came partly from herself – she'd decided that she didn't want to live like that any more – she had a wee boy who'd been taken into care, she had no job, no money, nae nothing, was just about to go to prison again. The work involved a lot of liaison, and cost a lot of money, but it was worth it because she's now got her child back, is in a full-time job, she's got a house and she's never offended since. That's a real success story. The whole process took about 2 years of work.

Of course, Arlon admitted there are failures as well, but she believes that as professional social workers, we should not dwell on those. She explains further:

Somebody said that working with the kind of people we work with is like trying to twist the lid of a sauce bottle – you can't do it, so you pass it on to someone else, and finally it'll come. So maybe sometimes you *do* make a difference, but you can't see it in the time that you're working with them. Sometimes problems are very deeprooted; sometimes people mature out of them; sometimes they don't;

sometimes it can take a long, long time which is outwith your span of work with that person, for you to see the results of your work.

In her work with drug users, Fiona is well aware that motivation is essential for success, but that this can be elusive, given the severity of some people's heroin addictions:

> You can get some people on the orders who are incredibly motivated, things happen, and it's gone – you try and get it back again, but if it's not there, there's nothing you can do. You hope that they retain some stuff that they've learned, so that whenever they are ready to do it again, they've got a bit more knowledge as to what's required, and that can help them, perhaps. I don't think it's wasted – it certainly gets them thinking about what they need to do – I don't think the problem has gone away, put it that way.

Creativity in probation services

In common with the UK as a whole, Scotland has placed emphasis in recent years on the development of cognitive behavioural programmes in prison and probation services, as a means of reducing reconvictions. While the effectiveness of such programmes is still being evaluated, it seems from early research that the majority of programmes *by themselves* are unlikely to deliver the outcomes that have been expected of them (Roberts 2004).

All the criminal justice social workers interviewed for this chapter stress the value of group work programmes as one method of intervention alongside others. They argue that intervention should always be tailored to individuals, rather than a 'one-size-fits-all' package. As Ron stated emphatically, the focus should always be on 'How can the programme be used to help you in your offending?', rather than 'Here is the programme that suits you'. Sarah manages the probation group work programme in Edinburgh. She runs a range of groups, including groups for men, for women and for those convicted of road traffic offences. She believes that group work is especially effective for this group, because, as she says:

> ... they are one of the hardest groups of people to work with on a one-to-one basis, because it's very easy to minimise – driving when disqualified and such – it works so well when you put a group of them together. We always ask for feedback from the groups, and folk say, 'I thought I was the only one who thought that until I got into the group and heard this and realised it was just nonsense.' Because we focus a lot on things people say to themselves to make it feel OK to drive.

Given the freedom to initiate a new road traffic programme, Sarah explored existing programmes before rejecting them as inappropriate for their client-group. As she explains, 'They were about the carnage on the roads – I thought that if you focused on the young joy-riding population, our 35-year-olds who drive without insurance were not going to make the connections.' So she set about creating an eight-session programme which would have practical aspects as well as more familiar, office-based discussions around a flip chart. She drew on all her ingenuity and contacts, and built a programme which now runs four times a year and involves the police and fire services, as well as social workers. The most exciting part of the programme for offenders is a trip to the fire school where fire officers simulate a crash, and then cut one of the offenders out of the wreckage.

What this demonstrates is that the group work programmes in Edinburgh currently use a mix of material from established group work programmes, as well as videos, clips from films, extracts from books, role play, discussions, trips out and worksheets which are completed by individuals. Hector admits that becoming a group facilitator as a relatively new social worker was 'very nerve-wracking in the beginning – in fact, going into every session is fairly nerve-wracking, till such point as the group becomes fairly comfortable and you become fairly comfortable with the material'.

It is worth noting that one of the reasons Sarah had to be imaginative in creating the programmes was because of a lack of financial resources for the groups. Only the men's group receives funding; the women's group and road traffic group are run on money carved out from the men's group work. The premises used for the groups are also far from ideal. The groups are located in a social work office at the foot of high flats, surrounded by graffiti and barbed wire. This is not a welcoming place to come, yet clearly good things can and do happen here.

An alternative approach: restorative justice

Niall works in a very different kind of criminal justice social work service: victim–offender mediation. Although there had been some small-scale schemes in the UK previously, restorative justice really took off after the UK government published a strategy document in July 2003 which called for its development for both adult and youth criminal justice systems.[13] This suggested that the aim should be to bring victim and offender 'into contact', direct or indirect, and this, for Niall, is helpful because it is 'do-able', and does not make greater claims than may be achievable. Niall sees mediation as a process which may or may not end with a face-to-face meeting. Whilst mediation was first used for what were considered relatively minor crimes, it is today being used with much more serious crimes, including, in one of Niall's cases, following a murder, when the parents of a young man who was murdered met the murderer following his release on licence into the community to ask him 'Why?'

Niall describes the work as follows:

> One of SACRO's key tenets in this work, the way we've been trained in this work, the whole theory of it as well, is to create a safe space for people to communicate. That space is not just physical, it's also psychological and emotional – my background fits very well within that. With a serious crime, we would take at least 6 months to prepare the parties to meet. We're exploring motivations, we're looking at the whole area of shame, guilt and how that can affect people – because that's part of the story – I would be bringing word back and forth.

Niall is aware that, as in all criminal justice social work, there are strongly political aspects to his work. He continues:

> There needs to be a lot of risk-taking to try different methods, in restorative justice and elsewhere. I worry more about politicians; that their policy is being dictated by what they read in *The Sun* newspaper or something – where you always see a punitive streak, and you don't get that more critical edge. Reoffending is a hugely complex issue, and no one intervention could ever claim to be, 'Oh, we got the offending rates down'. You end up running after red herrings to keep politicians happy. So what we're doing now is getting case studies together, promoting this as the voice of the people. But we're very wary of how we use the media, because they keep the perception going that the system needs to be punitive.

The work of SACRO, as a voluntary agency, is also highly dependent for its survival on contracts from government and some charitable donations. The mediation project is funded to take on 20 cases a month, yet the Procurator Fiscal's office[14] deals with 2,000 cases a month, suggesting that there could be far more use made of mediation than is currently possible. Niall believes that one of the reasons for the lack of funding may be the fact that the criminal justice system is 'offender-centred, not victim-centred'. His aspiration is that this might be broadened out in future.

LESSONS FOR THE FUTURE

As already stated, Ron has spent a lifetime working in social work services, and is therefore well placed to consider what criminal justice social work in Scotland might look like in the future. His overall assessment is that criminal justice social work has been driven by a narrow, political agenda which stresses the need to be 'tough on crime'. What troubles him most is 'the belief that by creating this gambit and plethora of interventions that you actually can cause crime to be cured'. Ron argues that what social work is good at – 'and charged to do' – may not be what the general public want in terms of criminal justice:

> We know why people commit crime – it's not because they're evil. Focus on their offending behaviour by addressing the welfare, pragmatic, practical problems that people have – is that what the public want? Because that's what we're doing, and are charged with doing. Equally, we're charged with supporting other social work colleagues attending case conferences where there are children involved.

It is interesting to note that some of the passion which Ron exhibits is also reflected in a recent review of criminal justice services (McNeill *et al.* 2005). This review argues that criminal justice social work is fundamentally about relationships with offenders; that criminal justice, like mental health, is a complex and, at times, messy field which cannot be reduced to technical, mechanistic interventions (2005: 39). Arlon expresses a vision for social work's role which is shared by many social workers and service users:

> We need to get into the community – to understand communities better. That bit of social work has gone – it's no longer part of our jobs. But I think it is. I think we need to get out there, building the links, strengthening communities, and working with the individuals on their offending behaviour. We need to be more aware of the part that communities play in actually producing and sustaining offending behaviour, particularly with the drug culture. A lot of the people that sell drugs, they don't actually cause crime, but they create the atmosphere where it becomes easy to commit crime – they are very often neighbours, but we really don't have any idea how these networks actually work. I think that's really important – *that* should be criminal justice social work.

ACKNOWLEDGEMENTS

With thanks to Bill Whyte and Susan Wallace from the University of Edinburgh for their advice and information and to Susan, Sarah Henderson and Niall Kearney for help in setting up the interviews. Also to Ron Lancashire for giving permission for us to meet staff and service users.

NOTES

1 Probation work in England and Wales is part of the National Offender Management Service (NOMS), which has responsibilities for both probation and the prison services. See http://www.probation.homeoffice.gov.uk In Northern Ireland, probation is managed by the Probation Board for Northern Ireland. See http://www.pbni.org.uk

2 See http://www.scotland.gov.uk/library5/justice/noswssgi-00.asp

3 SACRO (Safeguarding Communities, Reducing Offending) is a registered charity which aims to promote community safety across Scotland through providing high-quality services to reduce conflict and offending.

4 See http://www.scotland.gov.uk/News/Releases/2005/05/25113735

5 HM Young Offenders' Institution Polmont (formerly Polmont Borstal) houses young people aged 16–21 years convicted by the courts to serve custodial sentences.

6 'The Cruelty' was the popular name given to the Royal Scottish Society for the Prevention of Cruelty to Children (RSSPCC), now called Children 1st. RSSPCC inspectors were mostly men; they investigated cases of abuse and neglect reported by the general public. In 1968, the new Social Work (Scotland) Act gave responsibility for investigating child abuse to local authority social work departments and the role of the RSSPCC changed. See http://www.children1st.org.uk

7 The National Assistance Act of 1948 set up welfare departments responsible for residential care and help to older people and those with disabilities; most of this work was carried out by women (see Walton 1975). In 1968, the welfare departments merged with children's departments and health departments to become the new, generic social work departments.

8 HM Prison Castle Huntly is an open prison with capacity for 150 adult male prisoners outside Dundee, Scotland.

9 HM Prison Glenochil is located in Clackmannanshire, Scotland and holds long-term adult male prisoners in security categories. With a capacity of 496, prisoners can only be sent here from other prisons and cannot enter the prison system via Glenochil.

10 On 20 June 2006 the Justice Minister, Cathy Jamieson, announced that the system of early release of prisoners in Scotland was to be changed. Whilst 50 per cent would continue to be the norm for most offenders, sheriffs would be able to stipulate how long an offender should spend in custody before release into the community.

11 See www.scotland.gov.uk/Topics/Justice/criminal/16906/6826

12 This fits with Prochaska and DiClemente's (1983) stages-of-change model, which sees the change process as a cycle which begins with pre-contemplation, moving to contemplation, preparation, action, maintenance and possible relapse. At the pre-contemplation stage, it is asserted that the individual will have no commitment to change.

13 See http://www.restorativejustice.org.uk/Resources/pdf/Victim_Support.pdf

14 The Crown Office and Procurator Fiscal Service (COPFS) is responsible for the prosecution of crime in Scotland, the investigation of sudden or suspicious deaths and complaints against the police. See http://www.procuratorfiscal.gov.uk

REFERENCES

Burnett, R. and Roberts, C. (eds) (2004) *What Works in Probation and Youth Justice. Developing Evidence-Based Practice*, Cullompton, Devon: Willan Publishing.

Cree, V.E. (2000) *Sociology for Social Workers and Probation Officers*, London: Routledge.

Hough, M., Clancy, A., McSweeney, T., Turnbull, P.J. (2003) *The Impact of Drug Treatment and Testing Orders on Offending: Two-year Reconviction Results*, Findings 184, London: the Home Office.

Maguire, M., Morgan, R. and Reiner, R. (eds) (2002) *The Oxford Handbook of Criminology*, 3rd edition, Oxford: Oxford University Press.

McLaughlin, E., Fergusson, R., Hughes, G. and Westmarland, L. (eds) (2003) *Restorative Justice: Critical Issues*, London: Sage and Open University.

McNeill, F., Batchelor, S., Burnett, R. and Knox, J. (2005) *21st Century Social Work. Reducing Reoffending: Key Practice Skills*, Edinburgh: Scottish Executive.

Moore, G. and Whyte, B. (1998) *Moore and Wood's Social Work and Criminal Law in Scotland*, 3rd edition, Edinburgh: Mercat Press.

Newburn, T. and Stanko, E. (eds) (1995) *Just Boys Doing Business: Men, Masculinities and Crime*, London: Routledge.

Perlman, H.H. (1979) *Relationship. The Heart of Helping People*, Chicago: University of Chicago Press.

Prochaska, J.O. and DiClemente, C.C. (1983) 'Stages and Processes of Self-change of Smoking: Toward an Integrative Model of Change', *Journal of Consulting and Clinical Psychology*, 51(3): 390–5.

Raynor, P. (2004) 'Seven Ways to Misunderstand Evidence-Based Probation', in Smith, D. (ed.) *Social Work and Evidence-Based Practice*, Research Highlights 45, London: Jessica Kingsley.

Roberts, C. (2004) 'Offending Behaviour Programmes: Emerging Evidence and Implications for Practice', in Burnett, R. and Roberts, C. (eds) *What Works in Probation and Youth Justice. Developing Evidence-Based Practice*, Cullompton, Devon: Willan Publishing.

Scottish Executive (2005) *Statistics Bulletin CrJ/2005/8 Prison Statistics Scotland, 2004/05*, Edinburgh: Scottish Executive. http://www.scotland.gov.uk/Publications/2005/08/18102211/22156

Smith, D. (2004) *The Links between Victimization and Offending*, the Edinburgh Study of Youth Transitions and Crime number 5, Edinburgh: Centre for Law and Society, the University of Edinburgh.

Social Work Services and Prisons Inspectorates for Scotland (1998) *Women Offenders – A Safer Way: A Review of Community Disposals and the Use of Custody for Women Offenders in Scotland*, Edinburgh: the Stationery Office.

Trotter, C. (1999) *Working with Involuntary Clients. A Guide to Practice*, London: Sage.

Walton, R. (1975) *Women in Social Work*, London: Routledge & Kegan Paul.

Windlesham, D. (2001) *Responses to Crime*, Volume 4, *Dispensing Justice*, Oxford: Clarendon Press.

Chapter 4

Mental health
social work

INTRODUCTION

Mental health social work in the UK has undergone a period of immense change in recent years. The 1980s and 1990s witnessed the closure of many long-stay Victorian asylums and the development of community-based alternatives, as well as the emergence of a 'user movement' in mental health, at the same time as a rise in public interest in mental health and personal growth therapies (Campbell and Manktelow 1998). Change in the mental health world has continued apace in the 21st century, and the outcomes for service users and carers have been mixed. As the report from the Mental Health Act Commission highlights, the shift of resources from hospital to community-based services has resulted in increasingly understaffed, unpleasant wards which undermine the therapeutic purpose of inpatient admission (Mental Health Act Commission 2006). Moreover, the Department of Health and the Sainsbury Mental Health Centre have expressed concern about the poor treatment and care received by members of ethnic minority communities with mental health problems (National Institute of Mental Health for England 2003; Sainsbury Centre for Mental Health 2002). At the same time, research on social exclusion amongst people with a diagnosed mental illness has shown that the unemployment rate of people with mental health problems is around 75 per cent, the highest rate of any group of disabled people (Office of the Deputy Prime Minister 2004).

Mental health services across the UK are currently positioned between two competing policy imperatives. On the one hand, there is a move to de-institutionalise the community-based centres which were opened as replacements for long-stay psychiatric wards. It is argued that the needs of those with mental health problems are best met in mainstream activities; specialist centres are seen as stigmatised and stigmatising (Bell and Lindley 2005). The reality, of course, is that this may mean a reduction in what are already limited services for service users and their carers.

At the same time, attempts to change mental health legislation are pulling in a very different direction. Proposals for legislative change in England and Wales have sought to enforce compulsory treatment on those living in the community who are deemed to be a danger to themselves and others. Whilst this has led to the creation of an alliance[1] between service users, mental health professionals and the major mental health voluntary organisations to fight the proposals, the continuing concern of government to deliver on a 'law and order' agenda suggests this is an issue that is unlikely to disappear.

It should be acknowledged from the outset that the role of mental health social workers in the UK is unique in Europe. Social workers can be involved in the legal processes that result in decisions to detain people with mental problems in hospital. They also play a part in supporting service users in achieving recovery, assessing them for social care services and working with carers. Combining these activities is a complex task and there is ongoing debate about where social work fits in the changing mental health services (National Institute of Mental Health for England 2004; Care Services Improvement Partnership 2006). All of these tensions in mental health policy initiatives, their impact on social work practice and hence on people's lives, are vividly demonstrated in the interviews with service users, carers and practitioners.

THE CONTRIBUTORS

Most of the contributors to this chapter live in and around Belfast; one person lives in Edinburgh, and was invited to take part because of her work as a 'user consultant' to the social work programme at the University of Edinburgh. The Belfast contributors all share the unique experience of living or working in a city which, from the late 1960s until the signing of the Good Friday Agreement in 1998, was marked by the violent civil unrest known as 'the Troubles'.[2] Smyth and Campbell (1996) argue that there has been a tendency in Northern Ireland towards collusion in disregarding the ways in which conflict has affected social work practice in a society which is sectarianised. The Belfast contributors reveal the different ways in which the experience of living through 'the Troubles' has provided a backdrop to their daily living; it also, in some instances, can be seen as a major contributory factor in the onset of mental health problems.

The contributors to this chapter are four people who are service users, two carers and two mental health social workers.

Service users and carers

Helen

I'm a 49-year-old mother of three. I have been married for almost 30 years, and I am a carer involved in mental health services. I work part-time for a mental health carers' organisation, acting as a carers' advocate, running an outreach programme and a helpline and education training programmes for carers, and offering one-to-one counselling and support for carers.

Maggie

I'm 40, now working as a user consultant in health and disabilities in Edinburgh. I'm white and Scottish. I have three brothers and a sister. I'm not married, but I spend a lot of time and get a lot of pleasure being around my nieces and nephews – just like anybody else in life.

Mary

I am a mother of four, one girl, three boys, from Belfast, and I am 53 years of age. I have eight beautiful grandchildren. I care for my husband who has severe depression.

Sally

I'm a 43-year-old mother of three, separated from my husband. I was just discharged from hospital last month so I'm working my way back up. I'm very involved in the TELL group – that's Training, Education, Listening and Learning. It involves service users and service providers working together, because we feel we're the experts – we know what's best for our recovery.

Terri

I'm 27, single, no kids, a member of TELL and the Mental Health Alliance in Belfast, but I also do a lot of work with other groups outside, promoting awareness of self-harm. For example, I'm taking part in the National Inquiry into Young People and Self-Harm,[3] and I am also involved with the local Rape Crisis centre and Survivors for Justice, because these are the things I believe in.

Trish

I'm a 53-year-old mother of one. I had a career as a civil servant, then had to retire because of depression. I had a stroke and I have spent the last 10 years recovering. I'm very happy to be a member of the TELL group. I'm also a member of the Mental Health Alliance.

Practitioners

Ellie

I am a very busy team leader of a mental health social work team covering a population of about 120,000 people in Belfast. I have been in post for almost 2 years, but was a social worker for 15 years before that. I have two daughters who are away from home and I am very proud of them. I go to t'ai chi once a week to relax, and go to the gym a couple of times a week, and I'm in a rambling club. I do a lot of craft things, including renovating furniture, and enjoy baking and entertaining.

Gavin

I'm 34, male, Northern Irish, married. I am currently doing a PhD in Social Work at the Queen's University, Belfast, seconded from a post as team leader in an Assertive Outreach Team, a specialist mental health team for those that are reluctant to engage with services. My PhD is looking at how effective that service is compared with standard care. I am still doing out-of-hours work, working 'on call' one evening a week.

EXPERIENCING MENTAL HEALTH PROBLEMS

Before turning to discuss social work and services in general, all the contributors to this chapter said something about the impact of mental health problems on their lives and on their families. The themes which emerged all have resonance with wider research literature on mental health (for example, Barnes and Bowl 2001; Rogers and Pilgrim 2001), and reflect the idea that people with mental health problems are survivors, not just a bunch of symptoms or even a specific diagnosis (see Read and Reynolds 1996; Repper and Perkins 2003).

For Maggie, becoming ill was a shock for which nothing had prepared her. She puts this simply: 'I never knew anything about mental health problems until I had them.' Similarly, Helen's husband's mental illness hit her 'like a thunderbolt'. She describes the context of her husband's breakdown:

My husband had been under a lot of pressure through his job, and the pressure had been building. Living in Northern Ireland there were added pressures, from the situation and from his role as a manager of a social club. He had had experiences at the hands of paramilitaries, and this all added to the pressure of his job. For about 2 years before he became ill, I knew there was something. He wasn't handling things well, and something was going to give. But in my naivety, I always thought it would be his physical health, that he would have a heart attack or a stroke. I never in my wildest dreams imagined it would be mental health problems, because I knew nothing about mental health or mental health services.

Helen's ignorance of mental health problems and mental health services meant that she did not know what to do when her husband became unwell. As she relates: 'Even having to phone a doctor when someone wasn't physically ill was contradicting everything I knew, because he hadn't a broken leg or arm, and he wasn't throwing up, so why would we need a doctor?' But Helen's husband *did* need specialist medical help: 'He was totally beside himself with grief. He couldn't talk, he wasn't eating, he wasn't sleeping, he was just sitting on the bed, staring, and rocking back and forth. This was the beginning of my long slow journey into mental health services.'

Helen is picking up another theme here – that mental health problems are something which individuals and families learn to live with, rather than something for which there is always a speedy or easy cure. Helen's family doctor (her GP) prescribed Valium, and Helen hoped that her husband would quickly recover. But he did not get better, and was later admitted to the local psychiatric hospital, where he stayed for the next 8 months. Helen's three children were very young at this time (the youngest was just 18 months old). Thirteen years later, Helen's husband is still using mental health services, mostly on a day-care basis.

There are also issues about diagnosis, as Maggie demonstrates. She was diagnosed as having schizophrenia for 6 years before it was decided instead that she was manic depressive – now most frequently referred to as 'bi-polar'. She knew she did not have schizophrenia:

I knew this was wrong. But at the time, I didn't know how to fight to get anything changed on that. It took me a long while to convince people.

In talking about the carers' group which she runs, Helen suggests that actual diagnosis is less important than the effects of mental illness on people's lives, which may be the same regardless of the diagnosis:

'It doesn't matter whether the diagnosis is schizophrenia or clinical depression, the results are the same. The labels are not the true picture.'

For those living with and working in mental health services, ignorance and uncertainty are not the only issues which they have to face on a daily basis. There is also widespread stigma and distrust of those with mental health problems. Although Sally has found her sister to be a huge support throughout her illness, others have been less than helpful:

I have felt like a freak – you know, the name-calling – from neighbours – folk who are just ignorant of mental illness. We are now trying to break down some of the stigma, because people don't really understand – they are scared. Mental illness is so different to a physical illness, because a physical illness you can see, with your eyes – if you've a broken leg or arm. But with certain types of depression – you cannot see it; no one can see it. So it's hard.

Trish takes this further:

Even your family look at you differently, once you come out of the closet and let them know that you are suffering from some kind of mental illness. You see that slight wariness, slight distrust in their eyes, and they're not sure whether to accept what you say as being true, about how you feel, or whether it's just you fantasising – you're making it up. They don't understand – and some of them don't want to – they start to avoid you, you know? Well, if our own families do that, what chance do we have in the rest of the population?

Mary cares for her husband who has suffered for many years with serious depression, and has a range of physical problems including heart problems, arthritis, sciatica of the spine and diabetes. He has recently had a leg removed following a heart attack. She has experienced depression herself in recent years. Mary points out that although there is stigma about mental illness, mental health problems can happen to anybody:

Nobody wants to be sick – they'd rather be working or anywhere else – there's still a lot of stigma about mental illness, 'They're loonies, they should be locked up', but it could have happened to anybody, stress can just get on top of you. When it gets to the stage that you don't want to wake up, that's big-time serious – when you think there's nothing out there for you.

WHAT HELPS?

All the service users who contributed to this chapter identify family, friends and themselves as the keys to their survival and recovery. Over and above this, they have all had experience of different kinds of medical intervention, sometimes chemical (drug treatment), sometimes physical (electroconvulsive therapy) and sometimes psychological (individual counselling and group therapy). Social work has not always played a major role in people's lives, but where it has, it has been critically important.

Going the extra mile

The severe nature of Sally's mental health problems means that she has had experience of many different kinds and levels of care, sometimes acute, and at other times, more long-term. ECT, group work and medication have all been used at different times. Sally has had good experiences with social workers over the years. She now sees a social worker once a week and appreciates this, but would like to see her more often:

> My social worker is only a phone call away . . . She can see signs as well, if I am becoming unwell. I have built up this relationship with her so she knows – I have only to open my door and she can tell how I am for that day. She's also taken me out as well, because I have a phobia about going out, so she has taken me out for coffee – it's a good thing, it really helps me to get by. She really listens to what I have to say and does her very best if I need anything, like dealing with the Housing Executive, or dealing with a solicitor, things that I just feel right now I'm not able to do. She'll make phone calls on my behalf, or she'll help me write letters, help me word them, so she does quite a bit that I really value.

Sally's social worker is not just there for the good times, however. She has also been the person who, on one occasion, had to put in place systems for Sally's compulsory admission to hospital (known colloquially as 'sectioning'[4]):

> . . . she was involved once when I was sectioned, and stayed with me afterwards – she stayed back after hours – was still in my home at 9 p.m. that evening – so then the GP came and then I was sectioned. She took the steps necessary, thankfully, because I wasn't safe, but at the time I thought I was all right. That's the thing, that at the time, you're not aware of being not well. She rang the GP, rang my sister and the ball was rolling quickly.

This social worker has also recently introduced Sally to a behavioural chart, what she calls her 'wee planner'. Sally outlines how this works and why she finds it useful:

> I've homework every week. We've just started this recently since my last discharge from hospital, and it is good, because she asks me to set wee goals, but not unrealistic goals, and when I reach them, I give them a tick and myself a pat on the back. Say for example if I plan to come to the day centre, or plan to go to my daughter's, I write it down in the morning time – or ring my sister, or clean my bathroom – anything – and I couldn't believe it myself, 'What's the point in doing this?', but it does work, because when I did a wee task like this, and I ticked at the end of the day, when I was going over what I had achieved, I was surprised, so I was – so even the smallest of wee things can be important, so she helped me in doing this as well.

As a user consultant today, Maggie has different relationships with social workers now than in the past. When she was 'sectioned' 10 years ago, what helped most was that the mental health social worker took the time to involve her mother in the process, explaining what she was doing and why:

> She took me out to my mum's and explained everything to the both of us, rather than just trying to talk to me on my own. Now, she didn't need to do that, but it was good because me and my mum talked it through with the social worker and decided not to fight the section. This meant that I didn't need a lawyer, I didn't need to appear in court, so that was pretty good.

Maggie feels much more knowledgeable today about her condition and about the things which trigger her illness. She also understands why it is sometimes necessary for compulsory detention measures to be taken:

> Half of the time it's for my own protection – I lose control of time, and things like that – so I'm going for walks at 3 a.m. – and have no sense of road safety – I'm walking in front of cars – and I'm in a really confused state. But I've never been sectioned for being violent or argumentative or anything like that. It's horrible, because the only way you can get me back to normal is by using very strong drugs, and of course, using the drugs gives you all the side effects.

Maggie has clear ideas about what makes a good social worker. She describes the hospital social worker who has known her for years: 'she's friendly, you can talk to her, she's not stand-offish at all. If you've got an easy personality, that's actually half the battle.'

A cognitive behavioural approach

Trish has also found a cognitive behavioural approach helpful. She suffered from depression for years before experiencing a stroke 10 years ago. Now that her physical health has improved, she has been given support with her mental health. She reflected that it is not without irony that it took a physical breakdown – a stroke – for her to get the help she had needed for years with her mental health problems. A social worker from the brain injury team introduced her to a programme called 'the Path'. It begins by asking service users to identify their dreams. Trish outlines the programme as follows:

> To start off, they ask you, 'What is your dream – if you could have anything in the whole world for yourself, what would it be?' Whatever your dream is, that's up there. Then they look at more realistic things: 'Well OK, that's your dream, what is your goal?' There are seven steps over 9 months or a year – you work out the different steps and stages you need to go through to reach your goal or goals. My whole kitchen wall was spread out with these dirty great news sheets with all these different steps. It was really good, because it wasn't just me, and the team, it was me, my husband, my neighbour who's my friend (and also happens to be a social worker), Sheila, the deputy manager of the centre. So it's all the different people involved with you, either on a personal or professional level, who will help you and encourage you to go through your different stages. Then you all get together each month for a meeting where you talk about how you've got on that month: 'Have you done this or that?' It's a really good way of (not pushing) but encouraging you (and it is pushing a bit sometimes – you need that too – you don't like letting other people down). It gives you that incentive to keep on the right track, and keep doing the right things.

Trish admits that she never actually finished the programme – she began to resent the structured approach and rebelled against it – but she got as much out of it as she could possibly have. She does not have a social worker any more, but attends monthly meetings of the brain injury team as a service user representative, 'to show willing and give them my support because of the support they gave me'.

Whose side are you on?

Terri's account is very different, and begins with a damaging experience of social work intervention. Although she is now a young adult using adult mental health services, social workers first intervened in her life when she was 12 years old. She didn't, at that time, see this as positive; instead, she describes social workers as 'bombarding my life':

> There was a lot of stuff going on in the family, and I couldn't cope with this . . . and I got myself into all sorts of trouble. It ended up that one day I couldn't take any more. I took an overdose when I was 13, ended up in hospital and the next thing social workers were bombarding my life.

In thinking back over this time, Terri now feels that the social workers who became involved with the family took her parents' side; *she* was seen as the problem, not them. But what she was unable to admit at this time was that she was being sexually abused by a family member. Two years later, on disclosing the abuse, Terri was referred as an in-patient to an adolescent psychiatric unit, where she met a social worker who helped her for the first time. Terri takes up the story:

> It was the next social worker – the one in the adolescent psychiatric unit that helped me so much – she helped me find my voice. She helped me (I wouldn't say I can stand up for myself, sometimes I can and sometimes I can't, but without her I would never have been able to do it at all). Because I was angry, I was acting out. I'd have been quicker to hit someone than to say something to them. I didn't like being like that, but I just didn't know what was going on in my head, I didn't know what was going on in my life, everything was turned upside down.

What Terri found most helpful was that her social worker in the adolescent psychiatric unit accepted her story as true, and encouraged her to express her anger at the way she had been treated in the past. She supported Terri to take a complaint forward against her previous social worker, and to write an article for a social work magazine about the importance of knowing your rights. This was not an easy process, and in the beginning, Terri found it impossible to talk to the social worker; to trust her. She continues:

> I found it very hard to talk – she didn't mind – I used to sit with my back to her because I couldn't look at people when I was talking. But she just carried on talking to me and she got me out of myself.

The only way I could talk at the start was by pretending there was no one else in the room. Then I faced front but covered my face with my hair. It took me (I think it was 4 months) before I could look her in the eye – I would look and then turn away again – but it was just built up and built up gradually. She never once tried to rush me, or push me; she took it at my own pace. She was one of these people if you cried, she'd cry with you. I could never say a bad thing about her, because she and a teacher that was in school at the time (she had an interest in working with unruly pupils) brought me forward and got me out, between the two of them, they did an awful lot for me, so they did. I was even able to go on and hold down a job for a while, which I couldn't have done before. I worked in a crèche, then a café. I got involved in a group which ran workshops on kids in care – I ended up speaking in front of 100 people at the group's AGM. I was telling them how the project worked, and why it was so good. I was so nervous, but I could do it.

A few years later, I sort of deteriorated again, but that was to do with a lot of things, and it was nothing to do with the social worker. She wouldn't let me go; she was my social worker till I was 21, and then she had to give up, to give me to adult services. But we still kept in touch from time to time by phone. She's been through a lot herself – she's been very ill – but we still have that contact – she is the reason why I'm here, so she is.

Terri draws out two important ideas here. The first is that those using services appreciate it when someone is involved in their life over a period of time. This allows them to feel 'held' by the social worker – the social worker 'wouldn't let me go'. Terri's account also gives a clue that the relationship with the social worker became a two-way connection. The social worker had shared parts of her own life with Terri, allowing Terri to support her in a reciprocal way.

Preventive work or crisis management?

The service users and carers all recognised that help was often not available until there was a crisis; it is the crisis which makes a problem a priority for social work. This is in spite of repeated government assertions that preventive work is important and valuable (Office of the Deputy Prime Minister 2004).

Helen struggled for years with her husband's frequent hospital admissions and with her children, the youngest of whom was proving to be a 'real handful'. She eventually got help, but, as she recounts, 'not before there was a near disaster':

One night, she [the youngest child] was out playing and I was on the phone. My husband went to call her in to get ready for bed, and she ran the other way. He couldn't take it – he thought all the neighbours were watching and they were laughing; to her it was a wee game. He finally caught her and was very cross, and I put the phone down and had to come between them. I had to intervene to prevent her being hurt. I was so worried about my husband's state that I phoned his CPN [Community Psychiatric Nurse] to get help for him, and then all hell broke loose – child protection issues – alarm bells ringing – and I was thinking, 'But I've been trying to ring these bells for weeks and you haven't been listening.' So we were plunged into the middle of a case conference. There was police involved and everything – it was total over-reaction to my mind. We had the social worker from the hospital involved and he had to get a child protection social worker involved.

The case conference took place and there was no further action taken. The only outcome was that we attended a local family centre and I was given counselling by one of the social workers, and they had a playroom where they worked with our youngest child. The older two girls were also offered counselling, but the younger one just didn't want to know ... The social workers at that time concluded that we were a remarkably well-adjusted family, to be in such a disadvantaged situation, and that I was doing everything in my power to keep the damage to a minimum, and the kids were certainly never in any danger to start with, and the whole situation could have been handled a lot better.

Helen was grateful for the help they all received at this time. But she felt it was wrong that something like this kind of support had not been available at the start of her husband's illness to help the family cope with the illness and with the mental health system in general. Mary's experience echoes this. She has struggled for years with her husband's depression and deteriorating physical health and feels 'let down by the system'. Her experience has been that a long line of people have been involved with the family at different times, but that there has been no co-ordinated service, and no single person holding the work together. This is in spite of the fact that she describes her current social worker as 'brilliant' because she listens.

Self-help through a day centre

Three of the service users who were interviewed in Belfast attend a psychiatric day centre, run by the local hospital trust. It is located on an industrial estate on the southern outskirts of Belfast. The centre building was formerly the Grundig factory, making music albums, and some of the current centre users were employed there in the past. Because it was a factory, it has the advantage of being spacious and there is ample room for the arts and crafts and sports activities which the users get involved in. But a major disadvantage is the lack of windows and hence natural light. All three service users praised the day centre and its place in helping them to get better, and to stay well. It is also a place where they can be themselves without fear of stigma or abuse, as Sally explains:

> The day centre is a big part of my life and without it, life wouldn't have any meaning. Everybody that comes here feels the same – they don't feel any different to each other – so we can relax and feel comfortable with each other.

For Terri, the centre was a lifeline at a time when there was no provision for young people of her age. Even though a centre especially for young people has opened nearby, she prefers to continue to come to this centre where she is known. For Trish, the day centre offered a place where she could begin to recover from physical and mental illness in a safe environment. As she recounts, 'This was a wonderful safe place to do it. Nobody questioned me, looked oddly at me, they just accepted me for what I was at the time.' This acceptance allowed Trish to get better at her own pace. It has also enabled all three service users to make as much, and at times as little, use of the centre as they are able to. The centre employs only three paid members of staff; all others are volunteers, and there is a strong emphasis on service users helping themselves and each other. Trish explains:

> What I love about the day centre is the ethos of the place, where people are encouraged to take on responsibility for themselves, for the centre, for each other, and to work towards trying to change mental health services from the inside.

There is an important message here for those providing services. Day centres are being reviewed, and questions are being asked about the helpfulness of segregated services like this. But for the service users, specialist provision of this nature has allowed them to build their confidence and extend themselves in a secure environment.

BECOMING A SOCIAL WORKER

People come into social work for a range of reasons. Although there can be no single explanation, some persistent themes emerge. Gavin, in common with many others, chose to become a social worker because of what he sees as a mix of family and political reasons:

> Family influences were most influential for me. Both my parents were fairly public-spirited; service was valued in the house, and they were both a bit anti-authority and anti-sectarian. My father had mental health problems and tried to kill himself when I was about 17 years of age, at the time when I was consciously thinking about what I was doing. I was interested in politics – in change and positive change – and I worked for a year between school and university in night shelters in London and Belfast. I studied Politics, Philosophy and Economics at university, then did my social work training between 1993 and 1995 at the University of Liverpool, where Chris Jones and others in the radical social work movement strongly influenced my political philosophy.

Gavin's political perspective can, at times, make it difficult for him to reconcile his personal and professional selves. He acknowledges an 'ongoing tension about being involved in a system which you do think needs quite fundamental change'.

Ellie's experience as a parent and part-time community worker was equally influential in her movement into social work. She spent many years in voluntary and part-time paid work in her local community before having children and then while her children were growing up. She first worked with uniformed organisations (Cub Scouts and later Girl Guides), youth clubs and then went to work for the YMCA (Young Men's Christian Association), running netball, junior clubs, youth clubs, working as a summer school co-ordinator, training part-time youth workers and, latterly, running a women's group. This group was called New Horizons, and was set up to encourage women to move into education or work. Ellie explains what happened next:

> After my third year, I began to see great changes in this group . . . the members were moving on to do different things, and I thought – 'What am I doing?' My youngest daughter was about 14 at the time. I'd done various courses over the years, but I wanted to develop further. I phoned a friend and spoke to him about how I was feeling and said I was thinking about going into youth work. He said, 'What about social work instead?' I said, 'Don't be daft – I have no experience!' And he just laughed, and said put in an application form anyway. So I did. I was offered a place immediately and spent the next 2 years enjoying every single minute of it, devouring books, and putting understanding to a whole lot of stuff that I had done previously.

Living in Northern Ireland through the time of 'the Troubles', Ellie felt that the international ethos of the YMCA had a strong influence on her value-base:

> I liked it because of the international ethos of it – it was a cross-community organisation, it existed in lots of countries and it was inter-denominational. There is a Christian aspect to it, of course, but I believed we should keep the door open for everybody, offering basic food, shelter and acceptance – that was a big part of it. The centre took Catholic and Protestant children alike – there were no labels attached – and the YMCA did cross-community work before it was even thought about as such. All the young people were seen as potential young leaders, as people who had something to give back again. The YMCA also operates a programme called 'Friends Forever' where a group of young people travels to America each year, eating, sleeping and working together, and visiting each other's churches on Easter Sunday. I helped with this programme for 6 years.

It is these values which Ellie has sought to keep alive in her social work practice with people with mental health problems, and more recently, in her work as a team leader managing a team of social workers.

SOCIAL WORKERS DESCRIBE THEIR WORK

The two practitioners work in very different areas of mental health social work. Gavin works for an Assertive Outreach Team in the heart of Belfast; Ellie is based at a large psychiatric hospital which was built as a Victorian asylum in the countryside of Antrim in the late 19th century.

Assertive Outreach

The Assertive Outreach Team is a specialist, multi-disciplinary mental health service, which developed in the early 1970s in the United States in response to the issue of people repeatedly coming into hospital, settling in, becoming well, heading out from hospital and then only reappearing when they were in crisis again. 'The idea', Gavin explains, 'was to try and stay in touch with people to prevent that quite negative cycle from continuing.' Following a government report on priorities for action in mental health services (Department of Health, Social Services and Public Safety 2002), Assertive Outreach Teams were first introduced to Northern Ireland in 2003.[5] Gavin is aware that the service is controversial:

Sometimes it may be seen as a means of trying, not to *force* treatment, but to focus on medication compliance and to maybe change people, or focus on conforming rather than supporting people to avoid crises in the ways that *they* want to.

Even the service's name is contentious. Gavin said that his team do not use the official title usually, calling it the 'Community Outreach Team' instead, because 'it sounds like we'll be hassling people all of the time'.

Gavin outlined what it is like to work in a multi-disciplinary team where he, the social worker, is the team leader. He sees this as quite a radical departure in Northern Irish terms, because traditionally, the consultant psychiatrist has been seen as the most powerful person and the person who instructs the other mental health professionals. Although a team approach is used, where everybody is involved in everything, there is not as much blurring as expected. Each professional has their own area of expertise, hence 'the psychiatrist still prescribes medication; nurses are the only people administering medication; the social worker is the only person doing social work assessments; the occupational therapist's emphasis is on employment and therapeutic activity'. In addition, support workers provide help with living skills and building social networks in the community.

The clients of the Assertive Outreach Team all have what are defined as 'severe and enduring mental health problems', as well as difficulties in engaging with services, and they are people who take up a lot of community mental health workers' time. Gavin acknowledges that the term 'severe and enduring mental health problems' is problematic; not the most optimistic term to use. Specific diagnoses within this tend to be schizophrenia, manic depression, severe depressions, but not people whose problems are mainly related to addiction or learning disabilities or personality disorders.

The Assertive Outreach Team carries out an assessment – usually two workers do this together and then an individual support package is worked out for the service user. People may be seen daily, weekly or fortnightly; this varies according to what they need and are happy with. They may be seen by two, three and even four different workers at different stages. The idea is that everybody in the team gets to know the service user, providing more continuity with the team if someone moves on. The main objective of the team is to avoid compulsory admission, but Gavin admits, it does happen:

> ... and it's grim when it does – it can feel like a failure – the trust you have been building and working together can get knocked back a bit. It's always around an issue of risk – for example, self-harm,

attempted suicide – so it is usually clear that person is in crisis and there are sufficient risks to make it OK.

Gavin recognises that there are privileges for him and for the service users who are accepted onto the team's books. He has a protected caseload which is much smaller than that of conventional community mental health social workers; he is able to draw in other professionals routinely, without having to make the case for their involvement; and service users are seen regularly and often by a highly skilled group of specialist workers. (It should be noted that this is the very service which, as a carer and service user, Mary advocates, but has unfortunately been unable to access.)

A 'balancing act'

In reflecting on her long career in mental health social work, Ellie describes it as 'a balancing act'. Social workers have to balance competing needs of different family members. They also have to balance their own values and belief-systems with those of the people with whom they are working. Ellie chose one case to illustrate this, a case which she has often thought about over the years:

> In this situation, there was a mum, dad, two adult sons living at home in a house in a very poor condition. The GP had made a referral because he was concerned about the mum's mental and physical well-being. I was an energetic young social worker that was going to turn their lives upside down and bring about change. I did a home visit. The house was dire, there were a lot of animals about, walking over worktops and cookers, and the house really needed to be fumigated it was so bad. Mum was seriously unwell – she had a serious mental illness – and I tried to support the family to get the house cleaned up. Nobody worked – dad and the sons went to the pool room or wherever, leaving mum in the house on her own for long periods, and there was lots of alcohol about as well. Clothes were never washed; they were bought from a second-hand shop, and sat in the corner of the bedroom in a huge pile. There was never any cooking done – always 'take-aways'.
>
> Eventually I got the family rehoused, got their welfare benefits sorted out, got a washing machine and things, but when I went back to the house, the washing machine and fridge had been sold. I worked with the family for about a year and a half and then my senior said, 'Enough is enough.' The lady's mental state was deteriorating, and she needed to come in for an assessment. She came into hospital and remained for some time, and the nurses got to know her husband and take an interest in him, so that his needs were met as well. He

unfortunately had a stroke and died, so mum ended up in a residential home where she has flourished ever since.

Ellie went on to explain that this case worried her on many different levels. The woman's sons were furious that their mother had been taken into hospital, and accused Ellie of breaking up the family. They verbally abused her at their house and on the ward and made her fear for her personal safety. (Heightened anxiety about aggression in Northern Ireland made this a particularly scary experience.) Ellie suspected that their anger was, at least in part, selfish; they were unhappy that welfare benefits had stopped when their mother had gone into hospital. But she was also concerned, however, about her own intrusion in the family. Her standards of cleanliness and home care were clearly very different to those of the family, raising questions for her about 'What is OK?' A grown-up daughter, living away from home, has since reassured Ellie, telling her that she 'did the right thing – all that's happened was right'. But Ellie has been left with mixed feelings about the inevitable difficulties of intervening in people's lives. As she says, 'That's what social work is to me – balancing everything.'

Risk and protection

Gavin chose to describe a different situation, but one which was equally demanding for himself as a worker:

> I was asked to carry out an assessment on a young man who had taken a lot of drink and drugs and had wrecked his supported flat. He was very keen not to go into hospital. This felt risky, because he had clearly been very distressed leading up to the wrecking of the flat. By the time we had got there, he had calmed down and was keen to stay. He interacted with the GP and me quite coherently, explaining why he didn't want to go into hospital, and what he did want to do. This felt good, because in different circumstances, detention would have gone ahead and it probably would not have been helpful.
>
> With our support, he moved back in with his mum. He has been getting on OK. He is still very anxious about heading out – that's why he used drugs so much, to help him get out, but on this occasion, he'd taken so many, he was out of control. He's still very wary of medication and reluctant to get into that, which is also great to see. Legitimate caution, I think.

Interestingly, Gavin's comment suggests that he agrees with the service user that prescribed medication may not always be the solution for those with mental health problems. This view is expressed frequently in service users' accounts of mental health services (see, for example, Read and Reynolds 1996). He is also identifying the difficult boundary between protecting a service user and, at the same time, supporting him or her to manage risk. Real lives are never free from risk; good practice in mental health social work is likely to include encouraging service users to take risks so that their lives are more complete (Davis 1996). The task of social work is then to work in partnership with service users, carers, other professionals and members of society to ensure that the risks which are taken have positive outcomes (Cree and Wallace 2005).

LESSONS FOR THE FUTURE

All the contributors were asked to think about what lessons they would want to pass on to the next generation of social workers; what would make a difference in the future?

Helen provides useful feedback about the way mental health services can alienate service users and carers, for example, by using terminology that is not widely understood:

> At the start, I wasn't even aware who the staff were. There were a lot of initials bandied about – there was the CPN [Community Psychiatric Nurse], ASWs [Approved Social Workers], OTs [Occupational Therapists], and I didn't know who any of these people were and what their roles were. I was, by and large, left to find my own way about a system which I knew little about.

Asked what she thinks is important to pass on, she is unequivocal. She would like to put this question to all professionals in social care:

> When they are involved in delivery of a service, I would like to think if it was *them*, or someone they loved, is the service they give good enough? And if it's not, what can they do to make it better?

Maggie's advice is similar: 'Remember that you're dealing with human beings – it's not just your caseload – there's a name behind your case – remember little things like respect and dignity and treat the person how you'd like to be treated, or how you'd like a member of your family to be treated.' Mary echoes this. She says: 'When you meet someone, listen – treat them like a person, not a number. Let them know that what you're telling them really does matter, and that there is somebody out there willing to listen and to help. Social workers have to realise that they are a lifeline to the people that they're visiting, they really are.'

Helen has suggestions about what could make the service better. She advises that quite often in mental health, the focus is on the service user – 'it's as if their family are detached – they are a separate entity'. But family members, she urges, are all connected and what you do to one affects the other:

> So if my husband is not well, I'm not going to be feeling well, my children aren't going to be feeling great, even the dog doesn't feel great. You cannot separate people and isolate them. So if you're working with one individual, it only makes sense that you look beyond them and see who's connected to them. Who are they being supported by, who do they support themselves? And what other relationships do they have? Because they have to see the whole person, not just the condition they're presenting with, and not just in the surroundings that they're seen in. You need to join up the dots.

Helen's views are reflected in Jones's (2002) exploration of the impact of mental illness on families, where he argues that families ought to be considered more by those who make and implement policies in regard to people with long-term mental health problems. Helen points out that when one person is in crisis, others will need help too, and when a carer gets good support, then she or he will be better able to help the service user. This, Helen advises, is likely to help prevent the family breakdown which leaves so many people with mental health problems isolated and alone. Finally, Helen calls for social workers to take risks and to look at the big picture:

> . . . we are all so worried about making sure that everything we do is technically right, legally right, looking over our shoulders. You need to be able to step back and look at the big picture, and make sure that the service is as comprehensive as it can be. And not be afraid to take risks – because if we never take risks, we're never going to learn anything. No one ever got anywhere without making mistakes. I certainly hope I never stop making mistakes because that would mean that I'd stopped learning. Life's scary anyway!

As a social worker for 20 years, Ellie has a lot to say about where social work might be going in the future. She urges that social work stop and evaluate where it's going as a profession. She adds:

> When I was training, I had a real appetite for books and research. That gets lost when you come into practice, because you're so busy *doing*. Now that I am a team leader, I like to make space for social

workers to read – so that research does inform practice – this is the big thing for the future.

But there is something more. Ellie has struggled throughout her career in social work to hold onto her individuality and her creativity; this has sometimes led to frustration and conformation with management and structures. She explains her concerns for the future:

> In this *Agenda for Change*,[6] are we going to lose the creativity? Are we all going to become clones of each other, bureaucrats? Maybe this is inevitable in a time of transition, so that social work can get these bits right, but it must not be lost for ever. I'm also not sure that social work nurtures people enough. That's what I've tried to do throughout my life, whether with staff or with service users.

As a much younger social worker, Gavin has also struggled to hold on to something of himself in his career. One of the activities which he is most proud of is a weekly five-a-side football game he takes part in with service users and staff. He sees this as a very positive experience, allowing people to 'interact without the distance'. Most of the people who play are on Gavin's caseload, others have moved on or are back in hospital. Gavin and the other workers organise lifts to enable the service users to take part.

Looking to the future, Gavin argues that social work needs to value its role. He sees this as difficult for society because 'social work is characterised by grey and difficult issues where there isn't certainty and the clarity that people desire and value'. He continues:

> I think social work could be better at saying, 'This is what we do and it is really valuable, it's really difficult and that makes it valuable. This is necessary, but difficult, stuff and we want and need to do it.' In mental health especially, it's about moving away from the focus on risk to much more on recovery, rather than maintaining people and keeping people safe.

He concludes that working in mental health has been good for him too, 'because it forces you to think about yourself and your own mental health and your own self-awareness, and that's very helpful generally and it's important to acknowledge that I am definitely meeting my own needs – it's good to be aware of this and to be thinking about it'.

ACKNOWLEDGEMENTS

With thanks to Jim Campbell and Gavin Davidson from the Queen's University Belfast, and to the staff and users of the Derriachy Day Centre for their support in setting up the interviews in Belfast.

NOTES

1   The Mental Health Alliance comprises 77 organisations from across the mental health spectrum. See http://www.mentalhealthalliance.org.uk
2   'The Troubles' refers to the period of conflict in Northern Ireland beginning with the Civil Rights marches in the late 1960s and leading up to the political resolution enshrined in the 1998 Good Friday Agreement. Over the 30-year period, more than 3,000 people were killed, most of them civilians. (See Fay *et al.* 1999.)
3   The National Inquiry into Young People and Self-Harm was organised by the Camelot Foundation and the Mental Health Foundation, to report at the end of 2005. See http://www.selfharmuk.org
4   The term 'sectioning' refers to people being compulsorily detained under various sections of the 1983 Mental Health Act for 28 days for assessment (section 2) and 6 months for assessment and treatment (section 3). Mental health legislation across the UK is currently under review; the new Mental Health (Care and Treatment) (Scotland) Act 2003 came into force in October 2005.
5   Assertive Outreach Teams also exist in England and Wales. They were introduced to England and Wales under the National Service Framework for Mental Health. The Framework deals with the mental health needs of working-age adults up to 65. It sets out national standards; national service models; local action and national underpinning programmes for implementation; and a series of national milestones to assure progress, with performance indicators to support effective performance management (Department of Health 1999). For further information on the development of the model in the USA, see Stein and Test (1980).
6   See http://www.dh.gov.uk/PolicyAndGuidance

REFERENCES

Barnes, M. and Bowl, R. (2001) *Taking over the Asylum. Empowerment and Mental Health*, Basingstoke, Hants: Macmillan.
Bell, A. and Lindley, P. (eds) (2005) *Beyond the Water Towers: The Unfinished Revolution in Mental Health Services 1985–2005*, London: Sainsbury Centre for Mental Health.
Campbell, J. and Manktelow, R. (eds) (1998) *Mental Health Social Work in Ireland. Comparative Issues in Policy and Practice*, Aldershot, Hants: Ashgate.
Care Services Improvement Partnership (2006) *The Social Work Contribution to Mental Health: The Future Direction. A Report of Responses.* London: Department of Health CSIP.

Cree, V.E. and Wallace, S.J. (2005) 'Risk and Protection' in Adams, R., Dominelli, L. and Payne, M. (eds) *Social Work Futures*, Basingstoke, Hants: Palgrave Macmillan.

Davis, A. (1996) 'Risk Work and Mental Health', in Kemshall, H. and Pritchard, J. (eds) (1996) *Good Practice in Risk Assessment and Risk Management*, London: Jessica Kingsley.

Department of Health (1999) *National Service Framework for Mental Health*, London: DoH.

Department of Health, Social Services and Public Safety (2002) *Priorities for Action 2002/2003*, Belfast: DHSSPS.

Fay, M.-T., Morrisey, M. and Smyth, M. (1999) *Northern Ireland's Troubles: the Human Costs*, London: Pluto Press.

Jones, D.W. (2002) *Myths, Madness and the Family. The Impact of Mental Illness on Families*, Basingstoke, Hants: Macmillan.

Mental Health Act Commission (2006) *In Place of Fear? 11th Biennial Report 2003–2005*, London: the Stationery Office.

National Institute of Mental Health for England (2003) *Inside Outside: Improving Mental Health Services for Black and Minority Ethnic Communities in England*, London: Department of Health.

National Institute of Mental Health for England (2004) *The Social Work Contribution to Mental Health: The Future Direction*, London: NIMHE.

Office of the Deputy Prime Minister (2004) *Mental Health and Social Exclusion*, London: Social Exclusion Unit.

Read, J. and Reynolds, J. (eds) (1996) *Speaking our Minds. An Anthology*, Basingstoke, Hants: Macmillan.

Repper, J. and Perkins, J. (2003) *Social Inclusion and Recovery: A Model for Mental Health Practice*, London: Baillière Tindall.

Rogers, A. and Pilgrim, D. (2001) *Mental Health Policy in Britain*, 2nd edition, Basingstoke, Hants: Macmillan.

Sainsbury Centre for Mental Health (2002) *Breaking the Circles of Fear: A Review of the Relationship between Mental Health Services and African and Caribbean Communities*, London: SCMH.

Smyth, M. and Campbell, J. (1996) 'Social Work, Sectarianism and Anti-sectarian Practice in Northern Ireland', *British Journal of Social Work*, 26: 77–92.

Stein, L. and Test, M. (1980) 'Alternative to Mental Hospital Treatment. Conceptual Model, Treatment Program and Clinical Evaluation', *Archives of General Psychiatry*, 37: 392–7.

Chapter 5

Residential child care

INTRODUCTION

Residential child care was, at one time, 'at the fulcrum of services for children in need' (Department of Health 1998: 5). In more recent years, however, its fall from grace has been dramatic, damaged as it has been by a series of critical reports which have highlighted failings in the residential child care system (see, for example, Utting 1997; Marshall 1999), and research studies which have documented the poor outcomes for children who have been in public care (for example, Parker *et al.* 1999; Francis 2000; Barn *et al.* 2005). Recent reviews have identified poor physical health, mental health, educational and employment outcomes for this group (Knapp *et al.* 2005). Residential child care has become such an outdated concept that, as Smith (2003) points out, major social work texts which are required reading for social work programmes in the UK frequently do not include chapters on this.

Contributors to this chapter acknowledge that the low esteem in which residential child care is currently held has important consequences for those working in the field, and for young people themselves; that as long as residential child care is presented as a 'last resort', and 'the end of the line', its workers, and the children and young people who use its services, will also feel marginalised and disparaged. The chapter seeks to present residential child care afresh, by giving voice to some of the young people who have lived in the residential care system, as well as to some of the staff (qualified and unqualified) who have spent their careers working in the residential child care sector, in children's homes and residential schools.

We start with a point of clarification. This chapter is, as stated, about residential child care, not about 'looked-after' children. Children and young people who have spent time in residential child care in the UK are often called 'looked-after' children. This is something of a misnomer, since the term applies to *all* children who are supervised by a council when they are subject to a supervision requirement, order, authorisation or warrant under the provisions of the Children Act 1989 and the Children (Scotland)

Act 1995, or they are being provided with accommodation under the same Acts. Most 'looked-after' children and young people are, in fact, supervised at home, as our chapter on children and families' social work demonstrates. A recent report (Knapp *et al.* 2005) suggests that only about 11 per cent of children and young people in England and 6 per cent in Wales were 'looked after' in residential settings.[1] Most recent figures for Scotland (31 March 2005) suggest that 13 per cent of looked-after children were in residential accommodation;[2] the equivalent figure for Northern Ireland is 11 per cent (Mooney *et al.* 2004).

THE CONTRIBUTORS

Our initial idea had been to locate this chapter in Yorkshire. However, wherever we travelled in the UK, people offered to tell us stories about the impact of residential child care on their lives. As a result, the nine contributors live and work in Belfast, Darlington, Edinburgh, Huddersfield and London. Many of those who have contributed to other chapters also mention working in residential child care, because, historically, this has been a common route into the social work profession. At the same time, some of the contributors to other chapters have had the experience of being 'looked after'. As we noted in the introductory chapter, the boundaries between 'service user' and 'social worker' are not fixed, but change over time. Thus, two service users in this chapter have plans to undergo social work training in the future, and a third is already on a postgraduate social work degree programme.

Service users

Brian

My name is Brian, I'm aged 19, I live in Darlington. I now live with my mum, and I was 'looked after' and have been a care leaver as well. Currently I am working for a company called Investing in Children, which promotes the rights of children and young people. I have a modern apprenticeship with them, which means 2 days a week at college and 3 days at placement, and that's quite fun. I hope to go on to university to train to become a social worker.

Dannielle

I'm Dannielle, I'm 20 years old and I live near Huddersfield. I'm lively and outgoing and enjoy meeting other people. Social services first got involved when I was a lot younger, when I was about 4 years old. I'm on a training course now, to get me into work. I enjoy going out and I love looking after kids. My friend that I live with has five children, so I'm busy with children, but I love it.

David

I'm David, I'm 45. I grew up in London. There were seven children in our family; I am the eldest. My father was from Africa and my mother was from Ireland. From about the age of 4 years, I went into a children's home. I am now on a Master of Social Work programme and I have four children.

Sarah

I'm Sarah, I'm 24, I have a 5-year-old daughter and I live in Belfast. I am a project worker for Voices of Young People in Care, and train volunteers who are matched up with young people in the care system. I came to work here because I have the experience of care and I have the empathy and I felt that I could make a difference in other people's lives. I thought it would be really useful to apply my experience for something positive. I have applied to do an undergraduate social work degree.

Practitioners

Colin

My name's Colin and I'm 40 years of age, I've worked in residential child care since 1986. I qualified as a social worker in 1998, and I've been working at a 'close support unit' in Edinburgh for 13 years. I am now deputy manager. I'm married and have two children.

John

I've been working in social care for 20 years now and I could have qualified many, many years ago, but I decided to work with lots of different service user groups before doing my training. I've just turned 40, I'd set myself a personal goal of being a qualified social worker by the time I was 40, so I've achieved that because I've just finished my course and I feel really good about that. I'm a gay man.

Kathy

My name is Kathy, I'm 56. I have two sons, one who is 36 and one who is 39. I've got four grandchildren – two boys and two girls. I've been a single parent since my children were young, so I've brought them up single-handed. My children are very successful in their lives. I started working for Kirklees Social Services in 1986, and I've worked there ever since. I work in the Leaving Care team now.

Gayle

I trained and worked as a social worker in the United States before coming to London in the late 1960s. I have spent the last 35 years working in different social work settings in the UK. I worked for the last 2 years as an agency social worker in a Leaving Care team in London.

Mark

My name is Mark. I was a residential child care worker for almost 20 years. Before that, I had no real idea of what I wanted to do except some sort of vague desire that I wanted to work with kids, probably in an educational setting. In 2005, I moved from practice into teaching residential child care. I have three kids, aged 13, 10 and 8.

EXPERIENCING RESIDENTIAL CHILD CARE

Our four service user contributors have very different experiences of the residential child care system. This, in part, reflects changes in practice over time: the large children's home which David entered in 1964 does not exist in today's services. But the differences also reflect the diverse range of care careers which young people commonly experience, as research evidence shows (see Taylor 2004).

David and Dannielle were both small children when social workers first came into their lives. David remembers vividly the day when a social worker came to his house and tried to remove him and his siblings from home:

> I remember my mum lying in bed, and us children fighting the social workers, trying to stop them from taking us away.

David was just 4 years old, and, with his three younger siblings, he was taken to a Catholic children's home of 120 children. He was given no explanation for this move, but now believes that his mother had had some kind of mental breakdown. His father was a merchant seaman who spent months away at sea at any one time, and was unable to care for the children. David spent most of his childhood in two children's homes run by

Catholic Sisters, only returning home once to his father's care for about 10 months during that period. He remained in children's homes until he was 15 years of age, when he was informally fostered by a couple who lived near the children's home. David had become friends with the family. He had started doing 'odd jobs' for them, and, later, visited for tea, and they asked him if he would like to come to live with them.

David is acutely aware that the practice and standards of residential child care have changed in the years since he was living in a children's home. Looking back on his experience, however, he is able to place it within its time:

> There were people who really cared and that shone through; and there were people who didn't care and that also shone through. There were people that protected you, and people that abused you (and I use the term in the broadest sense). There was a nun who was the head of our children's home who was very, very fair, and kind, but not in a 'goody-goody' way – she was a just person, and she offered us protection. There were lots of things that I would criticise about that children's home, although I would say it was of its time, but she stands out as being a very protective figure. There was no under-standing of children's rights or children's voices at that time; we were at the mercy of lots of different forces – but she was a just person.

Dannielle also came into care when she was 4 years old, but, because of changes in child care practice, she was placed, not in residential care, but in foster care (see Waterhouse and McGhee 2002). Dannielle remembers social workers visiting her mother, and she speaks fondly of her mother's social worker who arranged her foster placement. Dannielle says she would like to meet her again, so that the social worker could help her to fill in some of the gaps in her childhood memories. Dannielle was adopted by her foster carers, and when she was 11, her mother, with whom she still had occasional contact, died. This death was quickly followed by another; her adoptive mother died when she was 13 years of age. Dannielle was subsequently abused by her adoptive father, and was removed from his house to a local authority children's home. Speaking about this, she said she was 'quite wary' when she was taken there, but her experience was OK. As she said, 'I was all right, because I was in my same school.' Later, when she started truanting and was finally expelled from school, it was the children's home 'key worker' and her social worker who 'helped me to get back onto a course – to get me back on track'. Dannielle is now living in a flat with a friend, but she has been back to visit staff in the children's home since she left; as she said, 'I go up when I can.'

The children's home in which Danielle was placed was very small in comparison to the home in which David stayed; there were only four children in the home. Nevertheless, Danielle is circumspect about whether a children's home can ever be a 'real home'. As she said with a wry smile: '. . . you can't really call it a home when there's an office full of files, and locks on all the doors.'

Unlike David and Dannielle, Brian did not come into care until he was 15 years of age, although social workers had been involved with his family for many years before that because of concerns about child abuse. Brian's mother had had severe post-natal depression so that when his parents were divorced, he went to live with his father, while his brother and sister went into a foster placement, before returning at a later point to their father's care. Brian is hugely grateful that social workers finally removed him and his siblings from home, because of his father's violence. He says:

> The biggest success for me was when I was actually removed from my father's care – when I was 15 – and at the time, my brother and sister and I were living with my father in County Durham. That was when times were really bad, because we didn't have any furniture, we were lying on the floor, he had the sofa, we had no cooker, there was never any food in and we had to go to an auntie's house to get fed. There was one night when I had to go to my auntie's to borrow a TV because ours wasn't working. My father had really beaten me that time . . . and my sister contacted social services and said, 'Look, he's been really beating us and I think it's time it stopped.' Social services came to my local school – a social worker who I'd never met before and a police officer came – they were very nice and I was able to tell them what had happened.

From that day on, Brian lived with different family members, including aunts and uncles and a grandmother, and even lived independently for a time. He is now back living with his mum, and is glad of her support. He has never lived in a children's home, although he has been a 'looked-after' young person, and he continues to receive support from an after-care worker.[3]

Like Brian, Sarah is intensely grateful that social services took her seriously and removed her and her sister from their parents' care. She is one of four children, all very close in age. Sarah's oldest sister had already left the family home and, with the support of a social worker, was living independently. Sarah takes up the story:

> Both my parents had alcohol abuse problems and home life wasn't good. There was a lot of physical abuse and things like that, but it

was more just due to the alcohol. It was actually myself and my other sister who found home life so difficult to cope with . . . We ran away, and went to my oldest sister. She had the name of an 'on call' social worker and she phoned her to say we were there. So the social worker came out and she seemed very shocked but she said she'd need to find us somewhere safe to go.

Sarah was clear even then, that with no extended family members to help her and her sister, she had no option but to go into care. As she says,

> We made the decision to go into care by ourselves. It was a big decision for an 11-year-old to make to go into care but it was the last option. Running away wasn't helpful, we'd no money, nowhere to go and nobody to stay with, so that was the only thing we could do.

Sarah and her sister were split up that evening, and placed in children's homes at opposite ends of Belfast. Sarah recounts: 'I remember sitting in my bedroom for a week and just cried. It was just the whole shock of everything that had happened and how fast everything had moved. And just being on my own.' Sarah also missed her younger brother greatly, and felt guilty at having left him behind. (Sarah said he had 'special needs' and was later also taken into care, after Sarah reported his neglect to the social services department.)

The next 6 years of Sarah's life brought mixed fortunes. She continued to live in the children's home until its closure 18 months later. At that time, most of the other young people in the unit were old enough to be placed in some kind of supported accommodation, but she was the youngest, and doing well at school. For this reason, it was decided that she should be fostered by the officer-in-charge, until another foster placement could be found in the same neighbourhood. Sarah spent what she describes as a very happy 6 or 7 months with the residential worker and his family, and then was placed with foster-parents for the next 2 years. Unfortunately, this placement was not a happy one, and Sarah was subsequently removed and placed with a single woman, who has been a main supporter and friend to her ever since. Looking back over her childhood experiences, Sarah is sanguine:

> There is lots of negativity about kids in care and social services, yet it has made such a difference in my life – I wouldn't be here today if I hadn't gone into care. I've used all my experiences to my advantage, and social services have played such a big part in my life and still do, as my friends, and I really appreciate how much they did for me.

WHAT HELPS?

Although the accounts here are primarily those of service users, it is inter-esting to see how often what they say is also picked up in the accounts of the practitioners.

One of the messages which was reflected in the accounts of both service users and social workers is that family remains a vital part of young people's lives, even when the impact of family members (and, in partic-ular, parents) may seem chaotic and, at times, destructive. So, for example, David was pleased that his mother and father visited him when he was living in children's homes, albeit occasionally, and that his father sent postcards from his travels abroad. Dannielle was deeply saddened by her mother's death, as was Sarah when her father died, even though their parents had been unable to care for them at home. Brian moved in with his mother when he was 17 years of age, after a lifetime of separation from her. The links he had retained with grandparents and aunts and uncles made this possible, in spite of his father's efforts to estrange him from his mother. And for all the young people interviewed, siblings played a key part in their childhoods, providing them with support, and, in Dannielle's case, fighting battles on her behalf.

Mark, a worker with 20 years of experience in residential child care, develops this theme:

> I think that families are fundamentally important to kids, even in situ-ations where we determine that being in that family isn't necessarily in that kid's best interests at times. I have worked with families that would be called 'dangerous families', but even in those families, they actually love their children, and in a strange way, they want the best for their children. So families are important – so if you *can* keep kids at home, you should do so. But then it becomes how you conceptu-alise residential child care – it is best seen as a *supplement* to family care, not an alternative to family care – there should be a partnership approach between families and kids . . . I believe that residential care should be seen as providing respite for families and for kids.

It is known from other research studies that young people like it best when social workers do ordinary things with them, treating them like ordinary youngsters, and, for example, taking them out to cafés (see Kay *et al.* 2003). Brian said that there was one social worker from social services who always knew when something was wrong with him:

> . . . she'd take me to McDonalds and we'd have chats there, she wouldn't bring a file with her, she wouldn't write notes, she was really

jolly, she wasn't patronising – that's one thing I can't stand, people who're patronising.

Dannielle agrees. She has contact with an after-care worker who has helped her with everything from health problems to housing, or as she says, 'Anything really. I see her every week usually, she comes to me. We meet up and go for a coffee.' But Dannielle is wise enough to know that in the past, she may not have always recognised the help she was receiving. She says:

> Social workers have helped me through a lot of stuff. I was too young to realise what was going on, if you know what I mean. They did help me through a lot of stuff, I probably wouldn't have been able to do it without a social worker – even up until now.

David makes a similar point. He puts it as follows:

> I am aware that there are people who make a contribution to our lives, and we never know what they do for us, behind the scenes. So Mrs B, who OKed for me to go into foster care – I will forever be grateful for that, but never knew what she had to go through to make this happen.

Dannielle admits that she has not always taken her social worker's advice, but she is always able to see later what the social worker had been trying to tell her:

> My social worker has always accepted what I've done, if she didn't like it, she'd tell me. I do listen to her most of the time, it's good advice they're giving you. I don't usually like taking advice, me, I think the only person I've really listened to is my social worker, because we've got a good friendship – I've always had a good friendship with her.

Dannielle is talking about something here which is reflected in all the accounts. The service users could all point to situations where someone had developed a relationship with them which the young person saw as a friendship, rather than a professional relationship. This friendship is demonstrated in two specific ways: in being prepared to 'go the extra mile' for the young person, even to the point of breaking rules (or at the very least, ignoring protocols), and in maintaining contact in an open-ended way, even when legal duties were no longer in force.

Sarah's story of her secondary school education demonstrates the willingness of a social worker to fight the system on her behalf. She had lost significant amounts of schooling when she had been living with her parents and looking after her younger brother. She needed additional support, and her social worker made this happen for her:

> My social worker helped me go through my work and broke every-thing down. I was struggling with Maths, but he arranged for me to have a tutor to help me through my GCSEs. I remember social services didn't want to pay for it, but my social worker fought with it and said I was making a lot of effort so you've got to give her it. And I ended up doing really well.

She goes on to relate what it was about her social worker that she most appreciated:

> I had a really good relationship with him. He was just excellent. If I had any problem, I could phone him at home. I wouldn't have phoned unless I really needed to and I knew that he would be there for me. Whatever happened, he knew me so well – he knew my history – I didn't need to say anything, he just understood and would do anything. He's still a very good friend of mine now.

Sarah's story reminds us that a good relationship can survive a crisis. She was placed with a foster couple who were part of a religious sect. She was deeply unhappy and the placement broke down, but she does not blame the social worker for this:

> Because I know his motives and it wasn't deliberate, and he made a judgement, although it was a wrong judgement. It's very easy to look back and say, 'Well, you should have done this', but it's very diffi-cult. I see him as a whole person, rather than just a social worker, and he sees me as a whole person, as opposed to just a case.

David also discovered the value of education, but in his case, it was his foster-parents who brought about the change for him:

> When I went into foster-care, I wasn't doing very well at school, in fact I was often playing truant, I was in a very low stream, I was just treading water. My foster-parents encouraged me to think of educa-tion as something which was really positive and valuable, and they wanted me to stay on at school, and I did so, and I managed to get three O levels. That might not seem a lot in the great scheme of things, but for me, that was a very big step, and set up an agenda for me so that later on I *did* go on to education.

As already stated, David was fostered because he was befriended by a local couple with whom he had become friends. He had been doing odd jobs in the neighbourhood, sweeping leaves and washing cars, and the woman was a teacher at his school. He gradually started to visit the couple and their children even when he had no jobs to do. Significantly, the resulting fostering arrangement was never formalised, because it was acknowledged by the social services department that it would be easier to proceed without this. As a result, the foster-parents never went through any selection or assessment process, and there was no preparation for David's placement. It seems unlikely that such an informal arrangement would be possible today, but this example shows just how helpful flexible support can be.

This is not, however, to suggest that social workers are not continuing today to find creative ways of supporting young people. Colin, for example, has continued to support a young man who is now 26 years of age, because the young man still needs him, although the residential unit in which he works has never before held on to a young person for so many years. Likewise, Danielle's after-care worker has supported her for 'the last 3 or 4 years'. As she relates: 'Because I've had her that long, we've built up a better friendship – I've got a brilliant relationship with her, it's really good.' Then she adds:

I don't even think I'm meant to have her now, because I was only accommodated in care,[4] I think I was only really meant to have her till I was 18, I'm not sure. But she's still involved with me now, and that's a good sign as well.

Service users did not only describe what they found helpful, they spontaneously offered stories of what had been unhelpful. Sarah gives one example:

So the next social worker arrived and hadn't read my notes. It was really rude and she was asking all these questions I'd never had to sit and go through before. I was really uncomfortable doing it and I did feel very much like a case to her. If we made an arrangement, she'd break it. We did actually get on very well, but she would say that she'd do something, and I'd have to chase her to do it. I did feel very much like a case to her . . .

Brian picked up another point:

Social workers who come into your home looking like a social worker, with a briefcase, or going to the school to pick you up – and I've had that – people ask 'Who's that?' And you try not to say anything, because people have stigma attached to them.

BECOMING A SOCIAL WORKER

Like the contributors to other chapters, social workers interviewed for this chapter had varied routes into the profession. Mark grew up in a family where both his parents had trained as teachers later in life, and it seemed inevitable to him that he would end up working in education, one way or another. Gayle did voluntary work with autistic children while she was an undergraduate student in the United States, and, although she never went on to work with autistic children, she believes it was this that motivated her to begin a Master of Social Work course in 1966. Gayle left without completing her studies, because she found the course too psychoanalytic in its approach. She later enrolled on another programme, this time at Howard, a predominantly black university in Washington DC. In her 40-year career, Gayle has worked in many areas of work with children and families, and has been a lecturer, trainer and consultant in social work, latterly working for a Leaving Care team in London.

Unusually, John was only 11 or 12 years of age when he decided he wanted to become a social worker:

> I think it stems from having a very large extended family – there were lots of aunts and uncles – and we had potentially every social problem going – it was interesting to grow up in that environment. It was about listening to different sides of the situation, and rather than being judgemental, it was about hearing and thinking, 'Oh, what was happening there?'

Although John had wanted to become a social worker from an early age, he did not think he was clever enough to do the training, so he went into catering instead. One of his first jobs was in a residential home for people with learning disabilities, and here he enjoyed the contact with residents and staff:

> . . . talking to the staff, they were just the same, ordinary people, not cleverer, not brighter, not any different than I was, so I began to retrain, that's where it started.

John spent the next 20 years working in social care settings, all the time increasing in confidence and skills, before finally beginning a social work course. Now aged 40, he feels 'ready' for the first time to be a qualified social worker.

Colin's initial entry into social work was surprisingly similar to John's. He recounts:

> I left school with absolutely nothing. I was happy to leave school, and had no idea what I wanted to do. I took a training course at college to become a chef, and I loved it. Then came the hotel trade and I hated it, the split shifts and the mad chefs. I went to work in a home for the elderly, then a job came up at St Joseph's, a residential school near my home. It was literally 10 minutes from my house; it was always called 'the bad boys' home' when I was growing up.

Like John, Colin found himself spending more time with the residential social workers and, of course, the boys. He played football with them and, with the encouragement of staff, gradually began to do shifts working with the kids, in addition to his catering shifts. He made the break from catering 3 years later when a post came up as a residential child care worker at the school. In 1996, Colin was seconded by his employer onto the Diploma in Social Work course at a local further education college. He did his first practicum (placement) in his own unit, which, he says, was difficult, being a student for half the week and acting assistant manager for the rest of the time. His second practicum was in a multi-cultural agency in another part of the city, and he 'had a fantastic time there'.

Kathy had a rather different life before moving into social work. She started working part-time for social services in home care with older people when she was in her mid-30s and a single parent, struggling to make ends meet financially. She also worked part-time for a building society doing insurance assessments, but when a 30-hours-a-week job came up nearer to her home, she applied for it and got it. This job brought her into children and families' social work; it was her job to go into families and help mothers to get children up and ready for school and then to bed again in the evenings. Some of the mothers were very young and struggling to parent their children; later, her work became increasingly with disabled children. When her own children left home, Kathy moved into residential child care, first into a small unit for four female care leavers, and later as a member of staff in a Leaving Care team, where she is working today. Kathy has completed the NVQ Level 3 award,[5] and more recently, the Diploma for Connexions Personal Advisers. This is an 80-credit course, validated by a higher education institution (in Kathy's case, the University of Huddersfield) as an undergraduate level II programme.[6] She has never gone on to do professional social work training; she worries she might be 'too soft-hearted' to be a children and families' social worker.

SOCIAL WORKERS DESCRIBE THEIR WORK

The government's Green Paper *Every Child Matters* (Department for Education and Skills 2003) heralded a new agenda which will bring organisational and structural changes to children's services in the future, as outlined in Chapter 2. The social workers interviewed for this chapter describe their work up to now and their own aspirations for future social work services with children and young people who have to spend time away from home.

Having fun with kids

Mark worked for many years in residential schools, in what were then called 'List D' schools.[7] The schools offered residential care and schooling to young people aged 12 to 16 years, most of whom had some sort of offending profile in their backgrounds, but, as Mark explained, 'this was not always the primary reason that brought them into care':

> I quickly came to terms with the Kilbrandon philosophy[8] that kids who offended or got into trouble, that their offence, or their difficulty, was actually a symptom of some unmet need. So I began to see that kids who offended were kids in need.

Mark's first job was at a school run by a Catholic brotherhood. He says that he found them 'inspiring – gentle and humane guys to work with'. They did not wear habits except on formal occasions, like for saying Mass:

> I learnt from them about respect for the individual, for the person, but also about discipline and about having fun with kids. Having fun with them has remained at the forefront of my mind, despite being expected to do social work with them!

Moving on to another residential school, Mark found the atmosphere there more bureaucratic and less pastoral. However, he remembers his time at the schools with affection, describing taking boys away on trips, cycling, hostelling, and, on one occasion in 1990, to the World Cup in Italy. Mark comments that such trips might be frowned on today as 'holidays for hooligans', but he saw them as a fundamental way of building relationships with young people, and also of giving the boys some of the good things in life. Just as controversially, Mark used sometimes to take boys home with him, first to his parents' house, and later, to his own home to meet his wife and children. He sees this as normal human interaction:

'I felt that this was one of the most powerful messages that you could give to a kid, that you were prepared to do that.' He criticises today's risk-averse culture:

> I regret that some of the more enjoyable aspects of residential care are not there any more, because of the risk culture that has emerged. I think this is concerning, because you are not talking about risk to kids, you're talking about covering organisational backs, and as a consequence, you are denying kids normal growing-up opportunities.

Since the 1960s and the anti-institution movement (see Goffman 1961), and because of financial constraints, the tide has swung decidedly away from residential care to family-based care, and many of the residential schools have closed down. Mark maintains that there will always be some young people who will do better by being away at school during the week. Recent research confirms this view (for example, Hill *et al.* 1995 and Smith *et al.* 2004). Mark is a strong advocate for residential child care:

> I think residential child care is still the best game in the world – if it's going well, and you've got a good staff group around you, it's superb, it's rewarding, it's great fun, there's an element of team work about it, there's an element of achievement, but more than that, it's that element of building relationships and making a difference through that relationship. The task of residential child care is about 'hanging out and hanging in' (Thom Garfat 1999)[9] – that encapsulates it very well ... and being there for them when things get tough and not rejecting them.

Supporting kids in care

Colin also began working in a residential school, then moved to work at a new, 'close support unit' in Edinburgh in the early 1990s.[10] Close support units (CSUs) were designed as short-term, intensive support units which would prevent the need for admission to secure accommodation and provide an after-care service for those leaving secure accommodation. To achieve this 'close support', staffing levels were higher than in traditional young people's units. In practice, it was found that the young people coming to these CSUs had so many difficulties that these could not be turned around quickly, and the units gradually became places that offered long-term support to groups of troubled young people, while they were in care and then beyond care. Colin explains this in his own words:

> We were working with some of the most damaged young people in Lothian, and we were saying – 'the buck stops here'.

One of the most telling stories which Colin recounted was about his decision to leave this unit for a promoted post, working for a housing association. He held the new post for just under a year, then returned to his 'spiritual home' at the CSU. The problem he faced at the housing association was that he was not allowed to 'work with' the young adults in his care; he discovered that offering 'housing support' was not enough for him, or, he believed, for the kids. Colin is still working today with a young man of 26 who came to the CSU when he was 12 years of age. Colin firmly believes that kids need long-term support and a steady influence in their disrupted lives; he describes one young person who came to the unit when he was 11, who had had 57 moves until that point in time.

Colin is not sure whether he is a social worker, although he has a social work qualification. He sees himself as a residential worker first, and suggests that the tasks he performs are complementary to those of social workers, but different. He strongly argues for the residential sector's being valued for what it does:

> Residential social work, for a long, long time, was viewed as a poor cousin of social work ... I'd like to think that it's not received as a last resort now – it's an opportunity to look at issues, work on issues, so that you can have what you want in life – it's not because you're unmanageable or at the end of the line. I think residential child care is now viewed (and should be) as a fresh start for young people, and the opportunities are there for them to meet their potential. Value the kids, value the staff, and you'll get that to work.

Supporting kids after care

Gayle and Kathy both talked about their work with 'looked-after' young people who had left care: Gayle worked in London, Kathy is still working today in Huddersfield.

Gayle outlines the context of her work:

> I was a social worker for young people between 16 and 21, but you mainly worked with the 16–18-year-olds. They had been in care and you were helping them get prepared to be young adults with education, jobs and accommodation.

She worked part-time, and with a small caseload of only five young people, she was able to see them regularly. Interestingly, she felt these young people faced exactly the same difficulties as the youngsters she had worked with at an early stage of her social work career, in Islington, in the 1970s:

They are still there with no money or support and the crunch issues are the same. . . . I spent most of my time, same as in the '70s, trying to get them places to live and most of what was there was bed and breakfast accommodation. You have to ask, 'How come they are still using bed and breakfast?'

Gayle noted that although there are more resources for after-care work today, bureaucratic systems are no better, so that there are often difficulties in getting young people the money they are due, and suppliers are still not paid on time:

You'd go to the department store and you would be standing with a kid who has hardly anything at all but has carefully chosen a bed or some knives and forks and they would say, 'No, you can't have it – your bills haven't been paid for two months, so we're not letting your London borough have any more.' You would think there is a way of breaking through this stuff, but it seems to be the same as it was back in the '70s.

Reflecting on her time with the Leaving Care team, Gayle added that

the most important thing is to keep close to the lives of people who need support. All the kids valued the talking time with workers. When other workers said to me, 'You seem to have time to talk with these kids', I'd say that you have to make time to talk to them because if you spend all your time just doing the paperwork or making the phone calls, it won't work anyway.

Kathy described her work in similar terms:

My way of working is – as long as I can do it – to put a lot of intense work in at the beginning, spending a lot of time with that young person. I find that if you put the work in at the beginning, when they're moving on to independence, you can slowly pull back and that's good for them . . . But as many times as they stumble and fall, we will pick them up and carry on and they can fall again – they're allowed to do that. And if their flat gets trashed, and they invite half the neighbours in, then we'll move them on, and carry on and they've got to be allowed to fall and you're there to pick them up again. Because that's what we're there for really.

Kathy feels that her job is easy because she knows what she is doing and, as she says, 'I know it inside out.' But what *is* hard is the unpredictability which comes with the business of supporting adolescents:

... it's hard in a lot of ways, because you have an island of calm where everything is fine, but you have eruptions where everything is 'in your face'. And all the time, it's how much work you put in, is how much you'll get back from the young people that you work with.

Kathy finds it impossible to operate simply as a nine-to-five worker, she allows young people to text her and call her on her mobile telephone. She thinks that is acceptable, because her family, after all, do this, and she is there for them. She adds:

And that's what we are – we're this corporate parent. I have my phone on from morning till night, unless I'm in a meeting somewhere, because I'm there for the young people, because that's what we're about.

John has just finished a social work placement working in a Children's Rights agency with 'looked-after' young people in Huddersfield. He says that what he has learned over his 20 years in social care is that whilst he is prepared to put 120 per cent into working with an individual, 'it's about where they're at, and if they're not ready to make the next step, then I think you can't push them'. He continues:

I worked with this young woman who was homeless and her mental health had deteriorated, she was having eating problems, she'd been raped, she'd been sexually abused, and we worked very intensively with her for 3 years, and managed to get her into psychotherapy, which threw up lots more problems and we were supporting her. We managed to get her into a 24-hour funded unit for people who've been sexually abused and she lasted a day, and this had taken months and months of negotiation. Rather than feeling really angry about that, it was about, 'No, she wasn't ready to do that'.

LESSONS FOR THE FUTURE

Asked about his views on how social work might support 'looked-after' young people better in the future, John was unequivocal:

It's about consistency, more than anything – what appalled me when I came here was hearing from the young people who said, 'Oh, I've had 13 social workers.' So what I'd say to student social workers is, if you're coming into children and families' work, come in for the long haul, rather than the short haul. At any age, young people need the consistency to find somewhere to unleash their emotions.

But something else is important for John, and that is not to think we have all the answers. He respects most the social workers who are still asking questions about social work:

> ... it's the ones that struggle with what they're doing and why they're doing it, whilst they've got lots of experience, they're still questioning what they're doing and why they're doing it, because they're so committed and they're so frustrated by the process and the way that departments and systems work – but they're still in there, because they want to make a difference.

Gayle observed that the social workers in her Leaving Care team were outnumbered by 'young people's workers': unqualified staff, who, like Kathy, did not have social work training, but might, or might not, go on to do it in the future. She saw these workers as 'more active and positive and less defensive than the social workers'. This connects with something Mark said, when he wondered if we currently train out of students the very qualities which they need to have for social work.

The young people interviewed for this chapter were very clear what these qualities are. Dannielle said:

> They've got to have good communication, be able to work with others, they need to be good at problem-solving, because you do get a lot of problems, good with children, being able to speak the truth.

Sarah came to the interview with a written list which she wanted to pass on, and she added to this in discussion as follows:

- Treat everyone as an individual – don't generalise.
- Take time at the beginning to read the file properly.
- Try to build up a relationship with someone before you start the heavy work.
- Listen to the young person – what they say is really valuable, and it can give them a lot of insight.
- Make your own judgement – don't rely on what the previous social worker said or what's in the notes.
- Confidentiality – I know there's a need to pass things on, but it's not good to go into an office for the first time and find that people know all about you.
- If you say you're going to give someone a service, give it and be realistic about it – if you know that you can't do something this week, but you can do it next week, then say that – don't just say 'I'll do it sometime', vaguely, and don't say you'll do something if you know you don't have the time.

- Be on time for meetings. It's very frustrating if someone says they'll be there at 4 p.m. and doesn't run up till 5 p.m. – you can then tell it's a whole rush, and the person isn't prepared and then they are worrying about their next meeting, looking at their watch.

Brian's views are similar, but with a slightly different emphasis. As a young child, he was unable to answer questions honestly when social workers visited his home, because his father was always in the room at the same time. He explains:

Sometimes the child or young person cannot speak out – the person in that room might be the problem – and if social workers can just try to get the young person away from home to talk to them, that would be great. Social workers should always ask a young person, 'Where would you like to meet and what time?' and not set up meetings themselves – always give them choices, and if you can't, always explain why you can't help them. But always keep trying. Treat the young person as an individual, and don't discriminate against them because they are looked after – so don't see them as a 'looked-after young person', but see them as a 'young person who's looked after'.

David agrees:

Social work has a responsibility – don't give up on people – it's really hard – there are lots of challenges, setbacks, closed avenues, but you don't actually know, in a way, the effect you're going to have on people's lives, but you do make a real, personal contribution to people's lives ... Our work on a local level can improve the lives of people by working side by side with people, getting into communities and supporting people to find their own voice – that's social justice – it doesn't have to be huge agendas, though they are important too.

ACKNOWLEDGEMENTS

With thanks to Rachel Balen from the University of Huddersfield and Maggie Speight from Voyage, Kirklees Children's Rights Service, for their help in setting up some of the interviews. Thanks also to Joe Francis and Mark Smith, the University of Edinburgh, for their suggestions on useful reading.

NOTES

1 Official Statistics and Surveys for England, Department of Health, at http://www.dh.gov.uk/PublicationsAndStatistics/fs/en
and Statistics for Wales, National Assembly for Wales, at http://www.wales.gov.uk/keypubstatisticsforwales/index.htm

2 http://www.scotland.gov.uk/Publications/2005/10/2791127/11278

3 The Children (Leaving Care) Act 2000 obliged councils to help care leavers who are subject to care orders until they are 21 years of age, and 25 if they are in further or higher education.

4 When a child is 'accommodated' by the local authority, this is a voluntary arrangement between the local authority and the family. This means that parents retain all rights and responsibilities for the child.

5 For further information on National Vocational Qualifications (NVQs), see http://www.qca.org.uk

6 For further information on the Diploma for Connexions Personal Advisers, see www.connexions.gov.uk/partnerships

7 Following the Kilbrandon Report of 1964, what had been called 'approved schools' were redesignated as 'List D' schools, because they appeared fourth in the Scottish Education Department's list of special education provision.

8 The Kilbrandon Report of 1964, as Smith *et al.* affirm, 'reasserted the primacy of a welfare and broadly educational approach to juvenile justice'. It 'identified the artificiality of any needs versus deeds split and prescribed education "in its widest sense" for troubled and troublesome youngsters' (2004: 61).

9 See http://www.cyc-net.org/cyc-online/cycol-0999-editorial.html

10 A recommendation that CSUs should be established in each Scottish city (Social Work Services Inspectorate 1996) was not subsequently taken up throughout Scotland. A 2001 report noted that there was no consensus as to what a 'close support unit' was and redefined 'close support' as a 'needs led, individualised package of multi-disciplinary intervention for young people in chaos'; see www.scotland.gov.uk/library5/justice/secureaccomint.pdf
The idea still exists today in Ireland where such units are called 'high support units'.

REFERENCES

Barn, R., Andrew, L. and Mantovani, N. (2005) *Life after Care: The Experiences of Young People from Different Ethnic Groups*, York: Joseph Rowntree Foundation.

Crimmens, D. and Milligan, I. (eds) (2005) *Facing forward: Residential Child Care in the 21st century*, Lyme Regis, Dorset: Russell House Publishing.

Department for Education and Skills (2003) *Every Child Matters*, Cm. 5860, London: the Stationery Office.

Department of Health (1998) *Caring for Children Away from Home. Messages from Research*, London: Wiley & Sons.

Francis, J. (2000) 'Investing in Children's Futures: Enhancing the Educational Arrangements of Looked after Children and Young People', *Child & Family Social Work*, 5(1): 23–33.

Garfat, T. (1999) Editorial, 'On Hanging-Out (and Hanging-In)', CYC-Online, 8 (September), www.cyc-net.org/cyc-online/cycol-0999-editorial.html

Goffman, E. (1961) *Asylums. Essays on the Social Situation of Mental Patients and Other Inmates*, New York: Doubleday.

Hill, M., Triseliotis, J. and Borland, M. (1995) 'Social Work Services for Young People', in Hill, M., Kirk, R.H. and Part, D. (eds), *Supporting Families*, Edinburgh: HMSO, pp. 119–34.

Kay, H., Cree, V.E., Tisdall, K. and Wallace, J. (2003) 'At the Edge: Negotiating Boundaries in Research with Children and Young People' [54 paragraphs], *Forum Qualitative Sozialforschung/Forum: Qualitative Social Research* [on-line journal], 4(2). Available [30-05-03] at: http://www.qualitative-research.net/fqs-texte/2-03/2-03kayetal-e.htm

Knapp, M., Fernandez, J.-L., Kendall, J., Beecham, J., Northey, S. and Richardson, A. (2005) *Developing Social Care: the Current Position*, Social Care Institute for Excellence position paper 4, London: SCIE.

Marshall, K. (1999) *Edinburgh's Children: The Report of the Edinburgh Inquiry into Abuse and Protection of Children in Care*, Edinburgh: City of Edinburgh Council.

Mooney, E., McDowell, P. and Taggart, K. (2004) *Outcome Indicators for Looked-after Children Year Ending 30th September 2002. Northern Ireland*, Belfast: Department of Health and Social Services.

Parker, R., Holman, B., Utting, W., Stevenson, O. and Bilton, K. (1999) *Reshaping Childcare Practice*, London: National Institute for Social Work.

Skinner, A. (1992) *Another Kind of Home: A Review of Residential Child Care*, Edinburgh: Social Work Services Inspectorate and HMSO.

Smith, M. (2003) 'Towards a Professional Identity and Knowledge Base: Is Residential Child Care Still Social Work?' *Journal of Social Work*, 3(2): 235–52.

Smith, M., McKay, E. and Chakrabarti, M. (2004) 'School Improvement in the Marketplace: the Case of Residential Special Schools', *Improving Schools*, 7(1): 61–9.

Social Work Services Inspectorate (1996) *A Secure Remedy: A Review of the Role, Availability and Quality of Secure Accommodation for Children in Scotland*, Edinburgh: HMSO.

Taylor, C. (2004) 'Social Work and Looked-after Children', in Smith, D. (ed.) *Social Work and Evidence-Based Practice*, Research Highlights 45, London: Jessica Kingsley.

Utting, Sir William (1997) *'People Like Us.' A Review of Safeguards for Children Living Away from Home*, London: HMSO.

Waterhouse, L. and McGhee, J. (2002) 'Social Work with Children and Families', in Adams, R., Dominelli, L. and Payne, M. (eds) *Social Work. Themes, Issues and Critical Debates*, Basingstoke, Hants: Palgrave.

Chapter 6

Social work with disabled people

INTRODUCTION

> We want to give individuals and their friends and families greater control over the way in which social care supports their needs. We want to support carers to care and individuals to live as independently as possible for as long as possible. We need to ensure modern care services are flexible enough to deliver support arrangements in partnership with others ... In the future social care should be about helping people maintain their independence, leaving them with control over their lives and giving them real choice over those lives, including the services they use.
>
> (Prime Minister's Strategy Unit *et al.* 2005: 7)

Mirroring some of the changes which have already been discussed in relation to mental health services, the past 40 years have seen a shift in the UK from services that offer disabled people segregated and devalued environments in which to live, to ones that promise them independence, control and empowerment in the community (Department of Health 2001; Prime Minister's Strategy Unit *et al.* 2005). This shift can be traced from the closure of specialist hospitals and residential units in the health and social care sectors from the 1970s onwards (Bornay 2005; Wistow 2005). Since 1990, the NHS & Community Care Act has transformed the roles of social service departments from service providers to assessors and brokers. As such they have been required to develop assessment and care management systems that act as gateways into the new mixed economy of care partnerships promoted by government as a more flexible and empowering response to user and carer needs. The introduction of the Direct Payments scheme[1] in 1996 pushed these changes further by enabling local authorities to make cash payments to some disabled people to purchase the care they needed themselves.

The changes to services and the role of social workers have also been shaped, since the 1960s, by the way in which issues of disability in the

UK have been politicised by the activities of disabled people's organisations. These organisations have campaigned for social justice, independent living and a voice for disabled people. Utilising the social model of disability developed by disability activists and academics, they have sought to influence policy direction as well as the education- and knowledge-base of social workers. This has meant that the dominant framing of disability as an individual, medicalised personal tragedy has been challenged by perspectives that have stressed the impact of social and environmental barriers on the lives of disabled people. (For further information, see Barnes and Mercer 2006; Campbell and Oliver 1996; Fyson and Ward 2004.) Social work education has been greatly influenced by these perspectives and the social model has become a basic tenet of its practice (Oliver and Sapey 2006).

THE CONTRIBUTORS

The eight contributors to this chapter currently live and work in a city in the English Midlands. Their experiences of disability and social work have, in part, been shaped by the ways in which the health and local authority agencies in that city have chosen to organise and reorganise the provision of social care and health services for disabled people over the last three decades. During this period these social workers, carers and users have found the social work services for disabled people continuously located and relocated in multi-disciplinary, specialist and generic teams. Most recently the social service department for adult social work services has been replaced by a new local authority department for disabled, learning-disabled and older adults, with a commitment to working for the enablement of individuals as well as the building of safe and secure communities for these service user groups. The organisational changes which have characterised the city's services reflect political and professional responses both to local and national policy shifts. Whilst each individual's account of the part that social work has played in her or his life is unique, they reflect some common experiences which relate to a shared, local context of service organisation and resourcing.

This chapter draws on the experiences of two people who are disabled, one person who is the parent of a learning-disabled adult and five social workers working in the local authority's specialist disability and learning disability teams. Like contributors to other chapters in this book, some individuals have experiences of simultaneously occupying other roles in relation both to services and to the education and training of social workers.

Service users and carers

Angela

I am a 46-year-old single female who is fiercely independent and has an acquired disability. I was a nurse before I got chickenpox encephalitis and became a wheelchair user in 1994. I am still adapting to people's changed attitudes towards me and I have gained a lot of knowledge of disability issues. I am not employed at the moment.

Helena

I work as a university resource administrator and I enjoy bingo, swimming and going to adult education classes. I was in a special school until I was 18 years of age.

Sian

I am a social work lecturer and the mother of two sons. My elder son, Michael, has Down's Syndrome. I was working as a social worker when I had Michael.

Practitioners

Cath

I am a white woman in my late 40s from a working-class background. I am a mother, a partner, a sister, a football fan and a social worker. I am someone who cares about people and cares about the world.

Emma

I have been a social services social worker since 1996. I work in a disability social work team. Before I became a social worker I worked as an au pair, a waitress, a cleaner and a care assistant. I am a vegetarian who enjoys red wine.

George

I have been a social worker for 28 years and work in a disability social work team that covers the south of the city. I am also a father, an allotment holder and a rock and roll fan.

Michaela

I am a part-time social worker in a social services learning disability team. I am a full-time mother. I have been committed to working with people with learning difficulties since coming into social work. I am a keen runner.

Phil

I have been a social worker in a learning disability team since 2004 when I completed my qualifying social work training. Before becoming a social worker, I worked as a support worker and advocate with people with mental health problems. I am a survivor of the psychiatric system.

EXPERIENCING DISABILITY

As disability activists and academics have argued, being born with, or acquiring, a physical or a learning disability means that an individual's identity is actively constructed by others, including those who offer health and social care services (Morris 1996; Mercer *et al.* 1999). This identity differs markedly from those around the individual and is characterised by difference, stigma, exclusion, loss of power and the denial of citizenship. It is then sustained through diagnosis and the social, welfare and economic arrangements that are made for disabled people by the society in which they live.

Angela's, Helena's and Sian's accounts of how they experience disability reflect these realities. For Angela, the acquisition of a disability in her mid-30s brought with it a life-transforming loss of independence. She was a nurse in the air force, enjoying the challenges of the career she had chosen and her independence as a single woman. In her 30s, she contracted chickenpox encephalitis which left her with substantial mobility problems. She had to leave her employment as a result. When she was discharged from hospital and returned to her home she found herself unable to manage life as she had in the past. She picks up the story:

> I was housebound, going round on my hands and knees and in a desperate situation. I had been in the Royal Air Force and had had to come out and I was at rock bottom. I decided I had to do something about it and I rang up social services to try and get some help, I asked to speak to a social worker ... I didn't see asking for social work as a positive, it was a negative for me – I did it because I was desperate. Getting a social worker got things moving though and it didn't take that long. The priority was to get the other services involved. They ensured I was getting all the payments; mobility, wheelchairs and access were sorted out.

But whilst this contact provided Angela with the basics she needed for re-establishing her life, she found that social work contact embodied a change in her situation which was difficult for her to come to terms with:

> As a result of getting a social worker involved the first time, the world and his wife came into my life and poked into every area . . . From being someone who was a very private and independent person I found myself needing the help but resenting it terribly – it was a love/hate relationship.

For Helena, receiving a diagnosis of being learning-disabled came out of the blue and set her life in a direction that she struggled to understand. The youngest of three children, she was 11 years old when she was told that she had a learning disability. She had attended her local nursery and primary school:

> I enjoyed going to school, it was ten minutes' walk from home. One day, they said my mum and dad had to come up to the school to see them. I was just about to go on to the secondary school. When my mum and dad saw the headmaster, he said that your daughter is slow at learning to read and write. He told them that because of the reading and writing, I would have to go to a special school. We had never heard of a special school before. They said to us they were schools that you had to go to if you were slow at learning to read and write. So I had to go straight there.

From Helena's point of view, the school she was sent to offered her no education at all. She explains:

> You just sat in the classroom; the teachers didn't talk to you. If you did something wrong you were told you were stupid . . . Everyone there thought we weren't worth anything.

At 13 years of age, Helena decided, with the help of her sister, that she would learn to read and write – 'I decided to get some books and do it myself.' When she was 15, she was asked to help out, unpaid, for 3 days a week in the school's nursery. But this evidence of her ability to work was not acknowledged when she left at 18 years old. In a final meeting with the headmaster, she was told that she would be going on training schemes for the rest of her life:

> I said I wanted to go out to work. He said, 'You can't go to work because you can't read or write.' I told him I could but he didn't believe me.

Disability arrived in Sian's life with the birth of her first son, Michael. He was born with Down's Syndrome, although it was not diagnosed immediately. She remembers being woken up in the early hours of the morning by a doctor who told her that on closer examination of Michael, who was in the intensive care unit, they had discovered he had Down's. She was then left alone until her partner arrived later that morning to visit her and his new son. She recalls remaining in hospital for a week or more while Michael gained weight in the intensive care unit. She relates:

> I was feeling very depressed after Michael's birth and I did not know which way to turn and was feeling quite guilty about some of the thoughts I was having about having a child with a disability and I really just needed someone to talk to. At the time, I was considering the options – alternatives to me caring for Michael full-time – I was thinking about the options of fostering and adoption and I just wanted to hear about them and have them offered even though I might never have taken them up.

WHAT HELPS?

In talking about what had helped them in managing disability in their lives Angela, Helena and Sian identified four key resources: their own efforts, the resources of friends and family, user or carer groups and, to a much lesser extent, social work. The relatively low profile of social work reflected the fact that for all of them, it appeared to be a scarce resource within the services with which they were in contact; social work was not offered to them unless they made a strong case for wanting it. For Sian, and to a lesser extent Angela, contact with social workers often delivered negative responses to their search for help and support. In contrast, Helena's first and only contact with a social worker provided the direction and support she needed to achieve major changes in her life.

Sian's contact with social workers was driven by her need to access services which she had heard about from friends and other parents of disabled children. She found that the responses of social workers to her requests for information about, and access to, these services were, in the main, less than helpful. Indeed on several occasions, she found herself involved in the time-consuming social services complaints system in her attempts to access a better response. She outlines how her initial request to see a social worker when she was in hospital after Michael's birth resulted in an exchange which failed to engage with what she felt she needed at the time:

It was a week after Michael was born. I am afraid that it wasn't a very good experience because the social worker came with her own agenda. She was obviously religious and she brought with her a little pamphlet that had been produced by the Down's Syndrome Association[2] and it was about the fact that I had been chosen by God – that my son was very special and I was a very special person and this was God's doing. It didn't go down at all well with me because I am not at all religious and it wasn't anything that I wanted to hear being said. So I effectively showed her the door and she never came back. After that, I don't recall having any visit by a social worker at a time when really I should have had someone to give me advice.

When Michael was 7 years old, and again when he was 12, Sian made contact with social services, asking about respite care and shared care schemes. On both occasions, she was seeking some additional support for the family in managing their life with Michael. This resulted in her accessing some respite care for Michael, but she felt that what was being offered left her and the family with other issues to resolve, as she outlines:

One of the things I was trying to avoid for Michael was him being in a segregated setting. But it seemed to be the only thing on offer, and in the end, I caved in to the idea even though intellectually, I was very opposed to it ... the place where Michael went for respite care was a segregated setting which confirmed all my worst fears of residential institutional care. The children were not treated as individuals – they were treated as a group. They went out in a minibus on outings which were not very stimulating experiences for them. It did give our family a break, but I was never convinced that it was serving Michael's interests.

More recently, Sian has found it difficult to access good enough social work input to key transitional review meetings organised by Michael's educational establishments. The social worker who attended Michael's review when he left school at 18 was a duty social worker with no knowledge of learning disabilities. Because of this experience, Sian fought for Michael to be properly represented at recent meetings at college:

Michael is nearly 21 now, and is in his second year at a residential college. He has a social worker at the moment. She is someone who works for the learning disability team. She was allocated as a result of us making a complaint to social services. We made the complaint because ... we were told that Michael wasn't entitled to a social worker and if we needed any support from social services it would have to be through the duty system.

Angela has found that she has been able, through her own efforts and the knowledge that she has steadily acquired through disability groups and organisations about services and resources, to maintain and increase her independence. But in doing this, she too has had to take initiatives and then keep the pressure on to get the response that she needed:

> No one actually informed me about Direct Payments. I learnt about them indirectly through various disability connections and I requested that I wanted to go on to Direct Payments. I wanted the control that the scheme seemed to offer. It had to go through social services so I approached them and then I had to wait. It was set up by someone who wasn't very sure about it and then there was a disagreement about whether I should make a contribution to my care.

This disagreement resulted in prolonged correspondence with social services in which Angela found herself quoting government circulars as she questioned the city's interpretation of the scheme. She eventually succeeded in moving onto Direct Payments in 2000 and was allocated a social worker. She valued her social worker greatly:

> I got an excellent social worker who I was very pleased with. She knew the system inside out and we got on very well and everything was working fine. We had a good relationship and I taught her a lot. We were on a level, she knew the Direct Payments system better, the paperwork and the bureaucracy and could work her way through it, I could come up with other things. We were open to each other and it worked very well. It was equal footing; I respected her as a professional and she respected me as a person who had a brain and could think and she was prepared to listen to me. It was a very positive experience. But then after a year, they decided that they didn't have enough social workers to stay with people and that I was OK with everything up and running and didn't need a social worker.

This has left Angela in a situation where she has had to regularly initiate and negotiate adjustments to her 'care package' with a changing array of social workers. Reflecting on her experience, she wonders how effective this way of allocating social work support is for both users and social workers:

> To get anything nowadays you need access. I can't do it directly – you have to do it through professionals. When you get a new social worker, they have to start afresh. You have to go through the same things, repeating them again and again. I'd rather be kept on the books of the same social worker and let them know if I had a problem so

they could pick it up and I wouldn't have to go through a 'getting to know them' phase and deciding whether I could trust them and where they are coming from. The way they do it at the moment seems to waste resources with waiting lists that take ages and it's not fair on new workers coming into a strange situation.

Like Sian and Angela, Helena's one and only contact with social work came from an initiative that she took. Aged 20, she had been offered two work-scheme placements which she found a 'boring waste of time'. With the support of her family, she had applied for jobs in local shops but she had not been successful. She decided that she was no longer prepared to stay on training schemes. When she announced this at the end of a day at the centre she was attending, she was told, 'Someone will have to come round and see you then.' She said: 'It worried me because I thought they'd send someone round to see me and tell me that I would have to go back.'

The person who visited Helena and her parents several weeks later was a social worker, called Alison, from the city's disability employment scheme. Helena found her approach completely different from anyone's that she had met before:

> She was the first one who was interested in us. We sat down and had a talk about my future and work and we told her what we wanted and what I would like to do . . . I felt good because it gave me confidence that someone wanted to know what I wanted to do.

Alison took Helena's desire to be employed seriously and helped her by supporting her to look for work at the job centre and linking her into a group for people with disabilities who were looking for work or were working. Through her support, Helena eventually secured a job placement as a part-time administrative assistant in a local university department. When Helena got this opportunity to work, she thought Alison would disappear from her life, but, as she said:

> . . . she stopped on. She said it was because she had to sort out my benefits when I went to work . . . She really knew what she was doing. I trusted her. She has always given me the right advice . . . She always had time to sit and talk. She was very good at explaining. If I didn't know something I could always ask her a question and she would always answer you.

After 3 years at the university, Alison suggested that Helena should ask about moving into a full-time permanent post. The suggestion surprised Helena but she trusted Alison, followed her advice and was successful. Six years later, Helena remains in a salaried job which has opened up opportunities for her to work as a service user, interviewing candidates for the programmes in social work. Helena has kept contact with Alison: 'I last saw her about 3 months ago to help me fill in a benefit form. She still helps me. It feels good knowing that she is there for me.'

BECOMING A SOCIAL WORKER

The five practitioners reflect the mix of backgrounds which characterise other social workers' reasons for becoming social workers.

It was a combination of religious beliefs and experiences as a service user that led Phil to become a social worker in his early 40s. He had been diagnosed as having learning disabilities at an early age and from his early 20s was a mental health survivor. Phil was fostered at the age of 13 months and experienced emotional and psychological abuse throughout his childhood from his foster-mother. He remembers the social workers who visited him:

> They conducted their interviews within earshot of my foster-mother. If they had conducted their interviews outside her earshot, they would have got a true and honest account about how I felt. I couldn't express my frustration about my childhood to anyone who would listen and who had the power to do anything about it. These social workers did have the power to do something about it and yet what they did was to collude with my foster-mother. They were just doing things as a tick-box to say they had done a review. They went through the motions.

It was not until his late 20s that Phil had a positive experience of social work. After a psychiatric hospital admission, he was allocated a social worker who had just completed her training. He explains:

> She was very nervous and she told me I was one of her first service users. I got a sense of her being accessible, good at her job and she handed over really well to a social work assistant who played a prominent role in getting me my first flat after my second breakdown.

These contrasting experiences, together with a decade or more of employment as a support worker with people with severe mental distress, led Phil to consider the possibility of social work as career. He visited a careers officer at the university where he was doing a research degree and was asked about his strengths:

> I said I was a person's person ... I had worked with people who had low self-esteem and low confidence and I was good at motivating

them, giving them a sense of hope, rebuilding their confidence, being a mentor to them, guiding them through alternative coping strategies. I said I had good listening skills. I was able to speak to people in ways that made them feel they had been listened to.

Phil was told that he was describing a range of skills that were 'a good match' for social work and, once he had been reassured that the 2-year training came with a bursary, he applied for a qualifying social work course.

For Michaela, Emma and George, the idea of becoming a social worker emerged in their teenage years as a result of a combination of family influences and opportunities to work with people through voluntary work. Michaela's cousin, with whom she was very close, was sent to borstal,[3] and this was a big shock to her and made her think about what she might do to help people. Her older sister was on a social work course and was able to tell Michaela something about what this might entail. Michaela subsequently finished school, did a year as a community service volunteer (CSV) worker[4] with disabled people and enrolled on a 4-year social work degree at university.

Emma remembers being interested in helping people when she was at school. 'I think I always wanted to do something in caring. When we were at school and we had a choice of doing something like sport or voluntary work I did voluntary work with what we then called "mentally handicapped" children in a hospital. I really enjoyed it.' On leaving school, she worked for a year in Germany as an au pair, started and then dropped out of a degree course in Languages and Business, and then combined waitressing and bar jobs with working as a volunteer on a telephone counselling service, because, as she said, 'I always wanted to do something helpful, caring and useful with people'. Emma applied to become an air hostess at the same time, but it took British Airways a year to call her for interview, and by that time, she had decided she wanted to do something in social work. She reflects on this:

If they had interviewed sooner, who knows, I could now be an air hostess with BA!

Emma got a job as a care assistant in a small home with people with learning disabilities, did a counselling course, and began a social care course at college. By the time she applied for social work training, it was what she saw as a 'natural progression', although she did not feel she knew what social work really involved at this time.

George recalled telling his school careers master when he was 17 that he wanted to be a probation officer. He had been brought up by religious parents, and describes himself as having 'lost the religion quickly but substituting it with a general wish to change the world'. He was advised that he could not train until he was 21 and was persuaded to go to university and do a law degree. This was not, in practice, what he wanted: 'I loathed and detested it from day one, largely because I felt like a fish out of water.' George was 'kicked out' at the end of his second year and became a CSV worker in a probation hostel in Devon. He found himself, at 20 years of age, being left at weekends in sole charge of men who had come out of Dartmoor Prison having committed serious offences. He says it was 'the most frightening experience of my life but it did give me a way into social work because I got a reference out of it from the Chief Probation Officer'. With this, he went on to get his first paid job in 1977, in a local authority children's home.

In contrast to these stories, Cath did not decide to become a social worker until she was in her late 30s. She left school at 16 years of age, and trained as a nursery nurse. When she was 20, she began nurse training, but quickly found it was not for her; she found the systems too hierarchical, and there was not enough time to talk to the patients. She went on to marry and quickly have two children, and began working as a nursery nurse at a crèche at a local college, because this was one of the few jobs which allowed her to take her young children with her. Cath progressed to working as a nursery nurse in a school. Looking back on this time, she said she knew she was 'stuck in the wrong career but couldn't afford to get out of it'. She did not know exactly what she was looking for, but she regretted that she had been unable to stay on at school, do her exams and go to university – this had never been an option for her. The Open University (OU) gave her a way forward:

> My husband went to work away, and I only saw him at weekends. I had no family close by so I was like a single parent really; there was me and my little girls. I started my OU degree. I was one of those classic people who got up at five in the morning, and I could do it – it didn't bother me at all. I'd work till seven o'clock and then get my girls up and take them to school in one road and I'd go to school in the next road where I worked as a nursery nurse. I did that for 9 years.

Cath sees this as a positive time in her life. Although she did not feel fulfilled in her job, the working hours allowed her to be there for her young children after school, and she enjoyed her Social Sciences degree. By the time her daughters were 12 or 13 and able to let themselves in from school, she began applying for jobs in social work, although at this stage she had had very little contact with social work, except as a very junior nursery nurse 20 years earlier, when she had worked at a family centre run by the Church of England Children's Society. Cath feels that it was her degree that led her into social work: it introduced her to accounts of social work practice and she thought, 'I'd like to do that.' She applied for a job as a social work assistant with disabled people, and was interviewed by a panel which included a service user. This was a valuing experience for her: 'I felt really comfortable at the interview, it felt right and I was offered the job on the spot.' Cath said that this was the job she enjoyed most in her whole career. She subsequently applied for a place on a social work course at the age of 40 years.

Working with disabled people

All the social workers interviewed made a positive choice to work with people who had physical impairments and learning disabilities. These choices were shaped by the contacts they had had with disability before and during their social work training.

Cath, as outlined above, had a job in a disability social work team before beginning her social work course. Reflecting on this time, she said that the people that taught her how to do the job were the service users:

> I really didn't have a clue, I didn't know what I was doing really and the service users taught me. They taught me about the Independent Living Fund, and that's where I got my real interest and love of it, and it began with one particular service user explaining it to me. So that is how I came into the job. It felt absolutely different from nursing. I was working with people and I loved every minute of that job.

On her social work course, Cath took the opportunity, through writing a dissertation, to learn about the new Direct Payments scheme. When she left the programme, she knew she wanted to work in disabilities, but her local authority had placed disability work into generic adult social work teams, which were dominated by work with older people. She negotiated a specialist caseload of disabled people with her team manager, as she explains: 'I came in so keen to do the work that I very quickly got it. I also said from the start that I was promoting Direct Payments and very few people on the team wanted anything to do with these, so I got the work because I was willing to take it.'

It was a 1-month residential placement with children with learning disabilities on her social work course that convinced Michaela that she had found what she wanted in social work. When she finished the course in the early 1990s, she joined a learning-disabilities specialist multi-disciplinary team. Michaela describes the team as follows:

> There was a sharing of understanding and tasks on the team. At that time, nurses did care management courses so they could do care plans

... You could ask someone to come out with you if you were unsure, as a one-off, and they would see whether they had anything to offer to support the person. It was a positive experience. I did more traditional social work tasks than I do now.

Phil had started his training course thinking he would work in mental health work on qualification, but his first placement in a learning disability social work team changed his views:

I discovered that often people who cannot speak for themselves are powerless and get a raw deal. There is a sense in which mental health service users are powerless and their discourses are marginalised, but people with learning disabilities are marginalised even more.

At a careers convention at the end of his training, Phil met someone who was a manager in a learning disability team. She was very positive about what he had to offer and he signed up to work with her team.

George moved into working with people with physical disabilities almost a year after he qualified in social work. For 3 years, he was a care officer in a home for adults with disabilities where a multi-disciplinary staff group worked to increase the independence of residents. After a spell in a mental health day centre, he moved for the first time in his career into field social work, joining a disability team in 1989. George has continued working with disabled people ever since, despite three major reorganisations of the service that employs him.

Emma moved to working with disabled people a year ago, following 8 years as a hospital social worker with older people. She moved into the area because she was looking for a change, wanted to work in a small specialist team and knew that some of her experience of working with disabled older people would be relevant to her new role.

SOCIAL WORKERS DESCRIBE THEIR WORK

In describing their current and past jobs, all of the social workers talked about what they valued and enjoyed about their work. All of them said that they valued the contacts with service users and carers; they felt they could make a positive difference to people's lives; and they had a positive regard for their colleagues. As Phil observed:

You get the feeling sometimes that people from a social work background are people you like – they appeal to you. I have colleagues that have empathic qualities and are really easy to get on with and chill out with. They say we don't choose our colleagues, but I felt mine had been hand-picked for me. I immediately felt that these were people who were good to be with.

An example of good practice

Emma, Michaela and Phil all used the word 'privileged' to describe how it felt to be allowed into people's lives and learn about who they were and what they wanted. Cath and Michaela said that it was assessment that they really enjoyed. For Emma, George and Phil it was the challenge of working out solutions to what appeared to be complex and intractable problems in the lives of users and carers. Michaela shared an example of the challenge and the pleasure that working with learning disabilities gave her:

A man, in his early 20s, who I got involved with, was placed in a residential unit. He had all these negative labels of having challenging behaviour and being aggressive. He had had lots of breakdowns in placements and this placement wasn't going very well. His parents were really supportive, but nothing seemed to be working. The team manager and I decided to go to the unit to do a little bit of person-centred planning[5] and most of the staff there were against us doing it ... When we explained that we wanted him to be there for the session, some of the staff said that 'he won't sit still for 5 minutes'.

But we were there for an hour and a half and he sat through it all and they were amazed. We got some really good information about his life. We asked him lots of questions – where would he go on holiday and what would his ideal holiday be? We built up a picture of him as a person. What was coming through the session was how he hated people invading his space, and he liked being on his own and yet he had been in residential unit after residential unit. We just thought, 'This can't go on.' We wanted him to try having a place of his own, and his family, thank goodness, were really keen to pursue this. This was key, because they were really driving it forward as well. So we went for it. He ended up in a shared ownership scheme. His mother helped him pick a property that was going to be ideal for him. He has a mortgage that he pays for through income support. He lives there on his own; he has 24-hour care, with two carers. The family are involved when it comes to interviewing carers.

Michaela went on to say that a lot of the problems that this young man had had in residential units (like serious damage to property) disappeared. She continues:

He has been involved in choosing the furnishings and everything. His mother has made it into a beautiful house. That is one of the best pieces of work that we have done. Pie in the sky it seemed to start with but we managed to achieve it.

Michaela reflected that as a result of this experience she had learnt a great deal about herself as a practitioner:

I learnt that I am prepared to take risks. I am usually a safe person; I go down safe routes. But if I really feel that something is going to work for someone I am prepared to take the risk and give it a go, even if I can't see how it has been done before and even if it hasn't been done before in that particular way. Someone else works with this person now and I ask about him. There have been hiccups – there always are, but he is still living in his own home and I think it's great, because of all the labels he once had, it must have changed his life so much.

Organisational stress

Whilst their work with service users is rewarding, the contributors all acknowledged the increasing difficulties that they were facing in delivering a service to disabled people and their carers. They described the disrupting impact of policy, organisational and administrative changes on their work, as well as the culture of management which prevailed. For example, Michaela graphically recounted the impact of the repeated reorganisations she had experienced since becoming a social worker. The first reorganisation led to the multi-disciplinary specialist team she had joined being dissolved after 2 years, and social work for people with learning disabilities being relocated in large generic adult teams. She relates the story as follows:

I found it a shock; it took a bit of adjusting to. Some teams retained their specialisms, but the team I went into wanted to have more of a mix. So you'd have a mixed client group which, in some ways, was very interesting. But in other ways, it wasn't. If I didn't have someone with a learning disability, I had this question about whether I really knew what I was doing. You felt like a jack of all trades and master of none.

After 6 months, Michaela volunteered to move to a smaller generic team where specialisms were being retained. But she found herself in a team dominated with older adult work, where the 'quick turnover' expected with older adults was inappropriate for the complex work she was undertaking with people with learning disabilities. She tried to negotiate a realistic workload with her manager and then decided she would have to reduce her working hours in order to manage the stress she was experiencing. Another reorganisation which re-created specialist social work learning disability teams seemed a positive move. But Michaela experienced the immediate change as 'a complete shambles. We had no desks, no phones and no computers. We had a room with nothing in and six members of staff – all social workers.' Because the team was understaffed, unallocated cases grew. Michaela now works part-time in a team where the duty system does not return calls for weeks, and new work is only taken on as the result of crisis or complaints. This leads to a very different kind of social work to the work she first undertook when she became a learning-disability social worker, as she explains:

> So it is very intensive work as soon as you get involved. The first step is often about building a relationship, because communication has completely broken down. It's not like any work I've ever done before. It feels like crisis work.

Phil, as a recent recruit to a learning-disability specialist team, confirmed Michaela's account of what is currently driving work in this area. In a team with lots of staff vacancies and over 200 unallocated cases, he has found allocation being driven by priorities relating to complaints, adult abuse and homelessness. In his experience, this means that: 'By the time people get social workers, they are in a bad way. You start by dealing with one problem that they want you to deal with, and then a whole can of worms opens up.' Because of this, Phil finds closing cases and moving on problematic.

Administrative systems

Practitioners were not, however, only concerned about reorganisations of services. They also criticised the administrative and managerial systems of their employing organisations, systems which reduced the time they spent with service users and created barriers that hindered their work on service users' agendas. In discussing these difficulties, the social workers echoed the views expressed by service users and carers about the lack of focus, continuity and responsiveness in current services.

Cath described the upheaval created by the introduction of a new computerised system, as follows:

> Compared to most social workers, I get on fine with computers, but I could not work this system out. It did not have any logic as far as I was concerned and that frustrated me immensely. We had to do care

plans on this system in a very rigid way. I was used to doing care
plans handwritten with the service user. Now the idea was that we
would do them at the office with rigid ways of entering things into
boxes. I found it very difficult – I hated it.

Like Cath, George is very committed to social work and to those with
whom he is working. He considers that given their background of working
with people who have physical disabilities, he and his colleagues have
imaginative approaches to their work and a commitment to promoting the
independence of service users. However, like Cath, he has found organisational initiatives difficult to accommodate in relation to his practice. He
explains further:

I really, in many ways, love what I do. I love it; I just hate and despise
the organisation I work for and it's never been able to produce
paperwork that does the job. It has never been able to produce appropriate paperwork and I think it is partly because it has lost sight of
what social work is. Or it no longer cares about what social work
is. I had this experience with being relocated with the reorganisation
12 months ago and there is a minor personnel issue that I have been
wanting to get addressed and I have made five separate contacts to
our personnel office and not one of them has been acknowledged.
So I have written to them, I have emailed them and no one has acknowledged my existence and, for me, that's a microcosm of how we are
viewed in the organisation we work for. We really don't count and
we are deeply unimportant and that makes me very angry. The paperwork has been produced, regardless of what social workers do, and
regardless of what social workers want. It's there because it's there
and I tend to use it as little as possible. I think that those of us
who have been in social work for a good while are confident enough
to go into people's houses and to gather the information that we
need and that we know what is relevant without using any of the
paperwork that we are told to use.

Despite these views George is still actively working to deliver what he
thinks disabled people and carers want, even if it conflicts with managerial priorities. His account of a piece of ongoing work illustrates what this
entails:

I have worked with a young man for 6 years, he is now 24. He got
a brain injury when he was 12. He is quite able physically, but the
damage has taken a great toll on his behaviour. He lacks concentra-
tion, he is extremely impulsive and gets into all sorts of problems.
Three or 4 years ago, he became a detained patient under a section

of the Mental Health Act. The hospital he went to was in another local authority area. Since then, I have arranged a number of placements for him. He has been in a private brain injury hospital, NHS psychiatric units and his own flat with support workers. All his placements have eventually broken down because he has done very well at first and then he has done something threatening. He is currently in a semi-secure psychiatric unit.

He is capable of independent living, provided that someone is prepared to do some structured, patient work with him on relationships and how he manages them, and that needs to be done in a structured setting. I know him and I know his mother and they talk to me a lot. I can give his history to other professionals quite fluently and I care about what is going to happen to him. I am very important to him and to his mother and they look to me to arrange funding for him because the NHS will fund anything that he goes to in the future. My manager says that it isn't our responsibility – we should close the case. But I have no intention of doing that, because if I did, he'd just be sucked into the mental health system where he is at the moment and they don't know what to do with him. He needs someone outside that system to try and get it to work a little bit for him. I need to stay put to do that, whatever the organisation tells me.

This suggests that practitioners have to be prepared to fight their organisations to give service users the support they feel they need.

LESSONS FOR THE FUTURE

These stories about the past, present and future of social work with disabled people contain a number of suggestions about how the approach that the government is currently espousing to service provision and social work practice can be achieved. Service users, carers and workers alike demonstrated that social work has an important and positive part to play in the lives of people with physical impairments and learning disabilities, particularly in relation to managing life transitions, providing information and advocating for resources. However, there was a recognition from the accounts that there is a growing gap between the aspirations of service users, carers and social workers and what is being delivered by services. All those interviewed felt that this gap had grown because of the ways in which organisations employing social workers are financed, organised and managed.

Practitioners, service users and carers highlighted the ways in which current levels of resources, as well as the organisational configurations and management styles of services, are failing to maximise the potential of social work. Lack of time for working with people, short and fragmented encounters with service users in crises and a growing and bewildering number of requirements around completing paperwork appeared to be the norm. In such circumstances, it is difficult for workers to work creatively and confidently and to acquire and use the knowledge they need in working with service users and their carers to realise choice, opportunity and independence in their lives.

The contributors also highlighted the uniqueness of social work in disability services because of its focus on meeting the holistic needs of people. This approach was found to be lacking in their contacts with the health and education systems. It was suggested that if social work with disabled people were to be more closely integrated with health services and delivered at a local level, it could result in more flexible and accessible services. But this will depend on social workers playing a major role in these services and there are strong messages about the kind of social work that is needed in the future for this to be achieved. Angela put this as follows:

> The key to good social work is openness and explanation. There is nothing worse than not understanding. You need to hear what is happening and why. It's also important to involve the service user where possible. You need to be honest when you don't know things. The ability to be able to think outside the box is a great asset. If you are working with disabled people you really have to think laterally. If you can't get round a problem one way, you need to find another way round it. You need to make sure that when you are helping people, perhaps less vociferous than I am, that they understand what is going on and are in agreement. If they are not in agreement, you must try to come to a solution that they can understand and feel a part of. Because it is other people's lives you are involved in, and you need to treat people with respect. Don't get so wrapped up in the bureaucracy that you forget this.

Helena was equally clear, based on her experiences, about what makes an effective social worker:

> Social workers should just sit there, listen to what people want, don't butt in when people are talking, and have some good ideas and good answers for them. Always use words that people understand, not words that they don't know, and smile and talk to people – get to know them. I know social workers are very busy because there are too few of them. But they have to make time for people and make them feel important and listened to, not look at their watch every 5 minutes and say, 'I've got to go, I've got to be somewhere else.'

Time was an issue too for the practitioners. All of them wanted more opportunity for direct work with people, for, as Cath expressed it, 'listening to people and spending time with people and enabling people to make a difference through completing detailed assessments with people and going away and making sure the assessment makes a difference to people's lives'.

In Emma's view, social work with disabled people 'has become very business-like, very much gate-keeping and not social work'. She said she believes it needs to be more personal and developmental, and less focused on process, meeting targets and the through-put of cases. She, like others, thought that a change in the culture of management and staff supervision is essential to support good social work. It was Phil's contention that this has to start from the top:

> The government must move away from quantitative measures of social work to qualitative. The tick-box culture is destroying social work. If social work is about helping people through transitions in life, people need time to articulate their needs and time to make decisions. And when you are working in crises, time isn't there and people are being left without time for choices.

ACKNOWLEDGEMENTS

Thanks to all the contributors for responding to our contacts and assisting us in the snowballing process.

NOTES

1 Direct Payments are cash payments made in lieu of social service provisions, to individuals who have been assessed as needing services. They can be made to disabled people aged 16 or over, to people with parental responsibility for disabled children, and to carers aged 16 or over in respect of carer services. The aim of a Direct Payment is to give more flexibility in service provision by enabling individuals to make their own decisions about how care is delivered, giving them greater choice and control over their lives. For more information see http://www.dh.gov.uk

2 The Down's Syndrome Association is a UK voluntary organisation which aims to help people with Down's Syndrome live full and rewarding lines. The association provides information and support for people with Down's Syndrome, their families and carers, as well as being a resource for interested professionals. It strives to improve knowledge of the condition and champions the rights of people with Down's Syndrome. More information available on http://www.downs-syndrome.org.uk

3 A borstal was a juvenile detention centre or reformatory, an institution of the criminal justice system, intended to reform delinquent male youths aged between about 16 and 21. The Criminal Justice Act 1982 abolished the borstal system in the UK, introducing youth custody centres instead.

4   Community Service Volunteers (CSV) is a UK voluntary organisation that aims to meet social need through promoting active citizenship and contributing to civil renewal. It has developed a range of volunteering opportunities in social care across the statutory, voluntary and private sectors. For more information, see http://www.csv.org.uk

5   Person-centred planning is an approach to empowering people with disability. Its methods and resources focus on individuals and their needs and put them in charge of defining the direction of their lives. It challenges service-led solutions and promotes the inclusion of disabled people as valued members of society. For more information see http://www.personcentredplanning.org and http://www.valuingpeople.gov.uk

REFERENCES

Barnes, C. and Mercer, J. (2006) *Independent Futures*, Bristol: Polity Press.

Bornay, A. (2005) *Disability and Social Policy in Britain since 1750. A History of Exclusion*, Basingstoke, Hants: Palgrave Macmillan.

Campbell, J. and Oliver, M. (1996) *Disability Politics: Understanding our Past, Changing our Future*, London: Routledge.

Department of Health (2001) *Valuing People: A New Strategy for Learning Disability for the 21st Century*, London: the Stationery Office.

Department of Health (2005) *Independence, Well-Being and Choice*, London: the Stationery Office.

Fyson, R. and Ward, L. (2004) *Making Valuing People Work: Strategies for People with Learning Disabilities*, Bristol: Polity Press.

Mercer, G., Shakespeare, T. and Barnes, C. (1999) *Exploring Disability: a Sociological Introduction*, London: Macmillan.

Morris, J. (ed.) (1996) *Encounters with Strangers: Feminism and Disability*, London: Women's Press.

Oliver, M. and Sapey, B. (2006) *Social Work with Disabled People*, Basingstoke, Hants: Palgrave Macmillan.

Prime Minister's Strategy Unit, Department for Work and Pensions, Department of Health, Department for Education and Skills and the Office of the Deputy Prime Minister (2005) *Improving the Life Chances of Disabled People*, London: the Stationery Office.

Wistow, G. (2005) *Developing Social Care: The Past, the Present and the Future*, London: Social Care Institute for Excellence.

Chapter 7

Social work with older people

INTRODUCTION

The 'ageing population' has become a major preoccupation for UK governments and policy-makers alike. Older people are living longer, and some older people are living longer in poor and worsening health. Phillipson (2002: 58) argues that the absolute rise in numbers of older people is less important for social work than the growth in particular groups, such as the very elderly (those aged 75 and over). He points out that in 1951, the percentage of the elderly population over 75 years was just one-third; it is predicted that this will rise to over 50 per cent by 2041. This is not, however, only an issue of increasing numbers of very elderly people. The falling birth rate, rise in geographical mobility and increase in women's paid employment mean that people (often, but not always, women) have less time and opportunity to look after their older relatives when they need care (Arber *et al.* 2003). Moreover, studies have shown that caring in mid-life has a range of adverse effects on employment and pensions of family members (Evandrou and Glaser 2004). Taken together, what this suggests is that greater numbers of older people require social work services now, and that demand for such services is likely to increase in the future.

But at this point, we must take a step back from the social policy 'facts' and ask: do all older people require social work services? The answer, of course, is 'no'. As Kerr *et al.* (2005) assert, age in itself is not a problem, pathology or indication of need; older people are not a homogenous group with a single set of needs. Many older people who come to use social work services do so because of the onset of illness or frailty in old age. Others may have had longer-term illness or disability which becomes more debilitating in their older years. In addition, the experience of old age, like all stages of the life-course, is governed by structural divisions of class, 'race'/ethnicity, gender and sexual orientation. Because of this, the choices and options available to some will be very different to those of others.

Successive studies have demonstrated that as a general rule, older people do not want to be dependent on others for help (for example, see Arber and Ginn 1992; Arber *et al.* 2003). On the contrary, they want to retain their independence as long as possible; staying in their own homes is by far the option of choice for most vulnerable older people. Yet, preventive services for older people remain underdeveloped and unavailable (Ray and Phillips 2002). The lack of services to meet the diverse needs of older people reflects, at root, deep-seated discrimination on the basis of age. Age prejudice has been around throughout history, demonstrated most acutely in the idea that termination of treatment may be advocated 'for the good' of elderly patients: Bytheway calls this 'the ultimate oppression' (1995: 27). The contributors to this chapter, each in their own way, challenge the ageism at the heart of current service provision, and urge us to develop more flexible ways of supporting older people in the future.

THE CONTRIBUTORS

All but one of the contributors to this chapter live and work in and around Bridgend, in South Wales; the one exception lives in Edinburgh and works in Glasgow. There was a strong sense from the Welsh contributors of their long-standing connections with the area; they were members of the community, whether they were using or providing services, and they felt a connection with one another as a result. Six social workers took part in this chapter, alongside four service users, two of whom were a couple.

Service users and carers

Harry

I am in my late 70s, have lived in Bridgend all my life. The wife and I got on all right together till she passed away. Then she left me in 2001 and it's been hard since. I have been in this bed for over 2 years now just moving between this and the commode. That takes me an hour and all my breath goes.

Annette and Brian

Annette said: 'I'm Annette and in a previous life I was a nurse and it has kept me in good stead in dealing with my present condition.'

Brian said: 'I'm Brian and for 33 years I was a policeman and it taught me one thing above all else – all policemen should marry nurses.'

Michael

I'm in a wheelchair all the time and I go out once a week on a Wednesday to get shopping. I have three sons a stone's throw away but they haven't spoken to me in a long while. I'm fiercely independent. I don't care, but it would be good to hear from the family.

Practitioners

Adrian

I'm 30, not married, I've been a social worker for 5½ years, have been working in Bridgend for nearly 4 years, and prior to that, I was in two other posts, both in neighbouring authorities. I was in hospital social work. My current post is with older people; I am now a senior practitioner.

Amanda

I'm a newly qualified social worker and a single mum of two girls – that's me, really, and family life with two children who are 11 and 13 years. Before qualifying as a social worker, I worked in the residential sector with adults with disabilities.

Dina

I am a social worker from India. I've worked in slums and educational settings and hospital and school settings in India and in this country, Scotland, with Women's Aid and I am now working in a statutory hospital setting with older people. I've been a social work educator in both contexts. I am currently doing practice teacher-training in Edinburgh, and throughout my career, I've had learning and teaching. When I was working as a teacher in India, I decided I needed further learning so came to Scotland to do a PhD. I am now again in the role where I might be a teacher. It's been a continuous circle of learning and teaching and things have evolved out of this.

John

I am a married man aged 60 who has been married for 36 years. My wife has recently qualified as a nurse at a mature age, as I did as a social worker. I have two children, a son and a daughter, both married, and 20 months ago my first grandchild came along and she is an absolute darling, the new light of my life. I am a bit of a sports fanatic and in my spare time I do sports writing for newspapers. I have had a varied career, I have enjoyed everything I have done but there have been times in my life when I have felt I needed a change and I haven't been afraid to do that.

Louise

I have been working for the same local authority since 1991. I started as a part-time clerk in an old people's home. When they started a scheme for older people with memory problems and their carers, I became their administrator, then they changed my job to become a home-care supervisor for the home-care part of the scheme. Then I became a community care worker in 2000 and then I applied to go on a qualifying social work course and I am now qualified as a social worker.

Suzy

I have been in social work for almost 5 years. After qualifying, I went to work in a learning disabilities team in Bristol, before coming back to Wales, initially to work with adults with disabilities. I am now a senior practitioner working with older people. I enjoy it very much.

EXPERIENCING THE NEED FOR SERVICES IN OLDER AGE

Asking for help can be a major hurdle for service users, whatever their age. Annette and Brian first received care services from their local social services department 20 years ago, when Annette became ill with a degenerative condition. However, they were very dissatisfied with the help they received at this time, especially from the carers that came to attend to Annette in the evenings, so they cancelled the service. This negative experience made them reluctant to ask for help again, and it was only because they were desperate that they were forced to seek help, as Brian explains:

> I physically could no longer manage my wife. As she got weaker, I got older and it became a real struggle and was dangerous. I envisaged us falling in a heap one night and being there for 4 or 5 days with a headline in the paper, 'Two old people found dead in Bridgend'. Annette had got to the stage where she was helpless. So we had to bite the bullet and go back to social services and say, 'Please can we have help?' and it was the best thing we ever did.

When they discussed the help they needed with a social worker she suggested that Direct Payments might be a way forward and provided them with information about the scheme. Annette and Brian talked it through together and Brian decided that it would add to his responsibilities as a carer and he 'didn't want the hassle of Direct Payments – perhaps 30 years ago I would have done it and thought no more of it, but not now'. So they opted for a care package provided by the local authority.

All of the older people who talked with us shared their frustrations at their frailty and asserted their need to hold onto personal autonomy and independence in spite of ailing health. Because of their illness and/or disability, they have to rely on others for help, either family members or paid carers and sometimes both. This can lead to feelings of powerlessness, lack of control and, at times, confusion and bewilderment. Michael expresses this well. He describes the way in which decisions are often taken on his behalf by others, and he is not always sure of the basis for these decisions. So, while maintaining that his carers are 'enormously helpful', he adds:

> I don't quite know how they attached themselves to me. I find them intrusive at times . . . They take letters away and they file them and they don't tell me why.

This illustrates vividly that the best intentions of a carer – to ensure that important letters are placed safely – can themselves lead to feelings of alienation in the person receiving care. It seems likely that best intentions were again to the fore in the decision to move Michael to a new flat:

> Someone took the decision not to put me back there [to his former home], and my own family put my stuff in this place. I came out of the institution and found myself *here*, not back where I belonged.

Of course, it is possible that the decision-making process was explained to Michael; that he unfortunately no longer has the capacity to remember the careful deliberations which took place before he was moved out of care and into his new flat. It is also possible, however, that, in common with the experiences of many older people, decisions were taken by others (relatives and professionals), and Michael was allowed very little say.[1] Dwyer (2005) draws attention to the power which others have over older people, and argues that social workers need time, skill, knowledge and values to facilitate a process whereby a service user can make up her or his own mind about the care she or he needs and wants.

Harry demonstrates that some older people can, and do, assert their opinions about what should happen to them, even in the face of the wishes of family members who have their own 'best interests' at heart:

> I tried the home once – the lads [Harry's two sons] thought it best after the wife died. They came and helped me pack the things and

took me there. They put me in a little room at the back, no view. I was sitting on the bed thinking 'I've got my own bed in my own house – why do I need any of this? Why am I here?' I rang the bell and she came in real 'la-di-da' and said, 'You should only ring that if there is an emergency.' I thought, 'Right, you can only have an emergency in here. I don't want that. I want a home.' I left a few days later and we had a meeting about what I wanted at home.

The package of services that has been supplied to Harry allows him to remain at home. But the care he receives is not all first-rate, as he will explain.

WHAT HELPS?

There is no doubt in Annette's and Brian's minds about the ingredients of good care. Annette says, 'The first thing is eye contact. It's important and so is manner – talking *to* people, not talking *down* to them.' For Brian, the key factors are having the 'right people' and training them adequately:

> ... they were the right people. They had been trained and knew what they were doing and it was a joy to be with them. Suddenly the house was full of laughter, they were the right people. They cared about what they were doing and they were communicators as well.

Harry also talks about the need for the 'right people'. He is prepared to accept that some of his carers are not the 'right people', but enough of them are to make it OK for him. As he says: 'I'd rather be here than anywhere and if it keeps me here, I'll put up with the naughty 'uns as well as the good 'uns.' He explains further what he means by this:

> Some of them don't care; they are not the right kind of people for the work, full of themselves and chattering. Do it in a few minutes, just in and out, it's like you're not there. Some of them are a real help, really genuine, listen to how you want it. Hugh's the best. He does the job properly and makes a cup of tea the way I like it done.

Harry is drawing attention here to the fact that conversation in itself is not enough; 'chattering' can be an imposition when it is one-sided. (Brian said something very similar, recounting that 'the odd one will just yak and forget to do some of the things'.) What matters to Harry is that his carer is prepared to listen and do things 'how you want it'. This takes us back to the familiar theme of autonomy and control. *How* a cup of tea is made becomes a marker of how far the older person feels that his or her life is their own; that he or she is still a self-determining adult. Autonomy and control are thus demonstrated in the ability to make choices. Annette argued that choice is very important to her too:

> One thing I can't stand is people saying things like 'come on now, flower'. I loathe it. When I was a nurse in the hospital, everyone was Mr or Mrs. No over-familiarity. You do get the choice in hospital. Now they do ask you what you want to be called. It's choice I want.

Michael makes a different, but related point; one which is also reflected in Annette's account. For Michael, it is important not only that carers talk to him and understand him. They should also 'pre-empt' his wishes, because when 'they are tuned in', he does not have to constantly ask or tell them what he wants/needs them to do. Annette said how helpful it was when carers anticipated her wishes:

> It was wonderful. I expected them to do things and they did and they anticipated what I wanted from them.

More than this, the carers made her feel as if she and they were all working together, as she said: 'It felt as if I was back on the wards again.'

Annette's husband, Brian, reinforced this message, but from the point of view of being a carer. Their social worker, Mary, organises respite care for Annette on a regular basis every year, to allow Brian to attend matches at Lord's cricket ground, in London. He picks up the story:

> She doesn't wait to be asked – she leads. She will say, 'Look, what about your cricket dates for next year?' and I have got them all written down and give them to her ... I don't get all the dates, but I get a lot. I can relax, enjoy myself and go to bed early.

From the accounts so far, it is evident that good social work with older people is about listening, genuineness and respect. It is about thinking ahead, and anticipating need. It is also, as Michael explains, about getting the balance right between risk and protection; between doing things for someone, and allowing them to do things for themselves:

> The carer group is enormously helpful. They get me up and put me into bed at night and they pop in to check up in between. They are my personal team and they are exceptional. They *want* you to be independent. I cook, clean, wash – not hoovering though – I do the

rest myself . . . I'm trying to get a wheelchair so that I can get out and go to the post office for 20 minutes where my granddaughter works.

Sometimes, care arrangements break down – a carer's baby is unwell, or someone is off sick. At those times, there needs to be a flexible response. Annette's and Brian's care manager has often stepped in when a staff member is off, and they appreciate this greatly. They have also welcomed their social worker's willingness to resource home adaptations which will support them: principally a hoist to help get Annette into and out of bed, and a clever technical device which Brian describes as follows:

> The vox box we have now is magic – do it all yourself at the touch of a button! We can put the lights on, TV, pressing a button and above all, it gives me my garden back, because it's a pager. For a long time, I never went out in the garden because if she calls me I couldn't hear her.

This example reminds us that social work services should support older people in various aspects of their lives, not just with personal care or relationships. This echoes one of the main findings of a recent study on effective social work with older people (Kerr *et al.* 2005).

BECOMING A SOCIAL WORKER

As in other chapters, social workers told different stories about their routes into social work. But, interestingly, all the social workers who contributed to this chapter talked about the importance of family experiences in their decision to become social workers.

Growing up in Mumbai, Dina felt it was something she was 'destined to do'. Her family home shared a wall with the College of Social Work, and every year, she went into the college for its annual exhibition. By the time she was 10 years of age, she knew she wanted to do something where she could 'help other people'. She picks up the story:

> I always knew that I wanted to work with people who were disabled in some way. So when I was in my early teens, I used to read to blind people and go into Mother Teresa's home for orphans on Sunday evenings. It was more of a public-spirited motive than a personal one. Soon after I finished my schooling at the age of 16, I went to do the next two years which would prepare me for my social work degree and then I did my five years' Bachelor's and Master's degrees in Social Work.

Amanda began social work training after her marriage broke up and she needed to 'stand on my own feet'. Her choice of social work was far from accidental. She had worked in residential settings with adults with disabilities before having her two children. Like Dina, she had been involved in voluntary work as a young person, this time through the Red Cross:

> ... we would take children, teenagers the same age as us with special needs and go away for a week, and have the most amazing time. It was fabulous! I suppose it was about looking beyond the disability and having amazing times and I've still got the photos and I look back over those times and it was wonderful!

Adrian said that he grew up knowing about social work. His mother worked in home care, and he identifies this as an important underlying reason for his decision to become a social worker. He did not immediately become a social worker, however:

> Social work was always something I thought about, even when I was in school, then I just drifted along and went off and did a degree straight from school, and then wasn't quite sure what I wanted to do after that, after doing the degree ... I applied for countless jobs in London and didn't get them, so decided to return home and I got a job working in the Housing Department in Bridgend.

Adrian worked in the Housing Department for about a year and, in this time, regularly came into contact with social workers, and, as he says, 'got involved in people's lives around their housing and wanted to get more involved with people and issues that they had'. So he applied for a social work course – 'and that was it'.

Suzy's mother had also worked in home care. But her reasons for coming into social work were more complicated than this:

> As a young person, I had a social worker myself and I got on very well with him. I didn't want to go into social work while I was at school – I was going to be a teacher. I went to teacher-training college but it wasn't for me so I dropped out. My mum had been involved in the social care profession as a home care worker so my understanding of what it was about came from there as well. After dropping out of college I did various jobs ... then I went to work in a nursing home as a carer – that's how it developed. But I couldn't start my training until I was 21 so I was filling in the gaps and getting bits of experience from everywhere till then. Then I did my training and haven't looked back.

Both Louise and John had very different careers before becoming social workers. She began in secretarial work and moved into social work after a time as a receptionist in a mental health centre. But Louise was clear that it was her close family background that brought her into social work. Her grandmother, who lived to be 92 years of age, had maintained her independence into her 80s, when 'memory problems' meant that she needed help from social services and medical staff. Louise worked closely at this time with the social worker and the community psychiatric nurse. She has recently joined the EMI (Elderly Mentally Infirm) team,[2] allowing her to specialise in work with older people with mental health problems, including dementia, depression and anxiety states and other psychiatric illnesses. Louise is determined that those she is working with get the same level of support that her grandmother did, in spite of their condition:

> What I like about the work is that you can make a difference. I think back to what my grandmother said years before she had memory problems, that she always had a strong desire to remain at home and keep her independence. I think that we can facilitate that – when people are vulnerable, keeping people for as long as we can in their own environment and promoting their independence. I want other people to have what my grandmother had.

John left school at 16 years of age with no idea what he was going to do; he went into insurance where he worked for 26 years. During that time, he thought about doing something 'entirely different but I was cushioned by a nice comfy 3 per cent mortgage, company car and a reasonable salary', so he stayed put. In the last decade of his working life in insurance, he and his wife set up an insurance brokerage and employed five people. But they found it was not what they wanted:

> ... it was totally taking over our lives. The children were grown up by then and I thought there had to be something more to life than this, really, and we made the decision to sell the business and I looked for alternative work.

John's sister-in-law had been disabled since she was 10 years old. She had had a stroke while undergoing a heart and lung operation. So from an early age, he had been familiar with the help she was receiving from social workers 'and it sparked an idea in my head that social work would be a possible interesting avenue for me to go down'. John sent off for an application form for social work training, while, at the same time, his wife applied to enter nurse training.

SOCIAL WORKERS DESCRIBE THEIR WORK

The social workers who contributed to this chapter work in hospital and community settings in the UK; moreover, Dina has worked with older people in India. Irrespective of context, all the social workers talked about the same things: about their commitment to those with whom they are working, and about their unhappiness with working environments that restrict the services they are able to offer service users.

Social work with older people in Mumbai, India

Dina's account demonstrates three features which resonate in the UK stories: the impact of lack of resources, the need for social work to be 'person-' not 'task-centred', and finally, the reality that social work is a 'last resort' service for most older people.

> Resources are very limited, with almost nothing paid for by the state. Because of this, there is huge pressure on social workers to find resources and stretch these, using these scarce resources for working towards some kind of amelioration of people's problems in these wide areas of health or education or communities . . . It was about finding the resources, stretching these resources, and using these scarce resources for working towards some kind of amelioration of people's problems in these wide areas of health or education or communities. A lot of time and effort was spent with people – a very 'person-centred', therapeutic approach was used; it wasn't task-centred at all . . . All these older people were destitute – generally a family, even when it is very poor, will hold onto their older members – but social changes – moving away from villages to the city – has created a large population of elderly destitute people.

The issue of resourcing social work services in the UK is very different to that of India. Our minimum expectations for nursing, social and personal care cannot, in any sense, be compared with the total absence of statutory provision in India. However, in both settings, social workers have to manage finite resources; and in both settings, they are confronted with service users' poverty. Johnstone (2002) argues that the shift in the last 20 years towards the privatisation of care for older people in the UK has increasingly led to social services becoming a residual service for poorer people.

'Safe discharge'

Moving people on from hospital to care in the community has been a major preoccupation of government in the UK at least since the NHS and

Community Care Act 1990. The Community Care Act 2003 goes as far as to force local authorities to reimburse NHS trusts in England and Wales in circumstances where a person's discharge from hospital is delayed because community services are not available. Dina works as a part-time social worker at Glasgow Royal Infirmary; the focus for social workers, as in all hospital social work with older people, is on 'safe discharge':

> To facilitate a safe discharge, the social worker is called upon to do a variety of tasks, ranging from having to clean the home, provide a bed – some older people have not been able to care for themselves and when it's time for them to go home from hospital, it is found that their homes are not really in a condition that is fit for human habitation.

Dina said she has been shocked by the living conditions of some older people with whom she has been working:

> I've had my baptism, if you like, by going into the first couple of homes that I went into in the east end of Glasgow which were completely shocking. There are people in this country, in the year 2005, who live on planks of cardboard, where there are plenty of resources available, who live in houses where there is no water in their pipes – they have been getting water out of the bathroom to cook in the kitchen; toilets and drains clogged up for God knows how long. These are some of the really desperate situations I have seen and where help has been needed to completely turn around the situation in their homes and make it fit for them to move in.

Task-centred or person-centred?

In reflecting on her current practice, Dina suggests that hospital social work is task-centred, not person-centred. It is essentially about assessing patients: assessing whether they can go home, or whether they can go into a nursing home, or whether they need another care package. She finds this work satisfying on the whole, 'because two plus two usually makes four – it does its job and requires immediate outcomes'. But Dina misses the intensity of relationships she was able to build with service users in her previous job working for Women's Aid. The expectation in her work today is that she has no more than two or three meetings with older people; she finds it difficult to provide the service which she feels that service users need within the parameters set for the job. Because of this, Dina regularly bends the rules: she spends longer with people than expected. As she says, 'in a way, I'm trying to find my own little niche in the way I want to practise'.

Asked to describe a case where she felt she made a difference with a service user, Dina gave the following account:

> This is the case of a 65-year-old woman, I'll call her Ellen. She had had a stroke which left her badly paralysed. She was slowly regaining use of her left side when she was diagnosed with breast cancer. She took that really badly; she had to have an immediate mastectomy. Over time, it became increasingly clear that she could not go back home, but she was very keen to go back home because she has a daughter who is 27 who has cystic fibrosis, and she's been the main carer for her daughter. (She was divorced from her husband when the child was only 2 years old.) She was afraid that if she went into care, her home would be taken away in lieu of payments for her nursing home. She was extremely distressed and her recovery was rather slow as a result. She was put into an ancillary hospital and when I first met her, she was extremely depressed and I spent 2½ hours with her and she told me her life story. I carried out a comprehensive assessment with her – I see this as a holistic tool, though some social workers don't like it – I like trying to understand a person not just in an intake kind of way, but in a more holistic way. I found the tool very useful, as an interview guide to help me understand the person. In going to see her, I felt as if I was going in to interview a woman about her life, and I felt very comfortable in this role, though it was surprising to the nurses and to the practice team manager that I was spending the first three sessions with someone who was crying and telling me about her life.

In carrying out the assessment, Dina also spoke to Ellen's sister, and to her daughter, and went on to make a strong case in writing for Ellen's home not being taken into account in deciding the level of fees she would have to pay for her care. Dina's last task was to take Ellen to visit possible nursing homes:

> So we made appointments in seven different homes, booked a taxi and packed a lunch, and the last home was the best one. Ellen felt she could feel comfortable there – she's now been there for the last 2 weeks and is already fairly settled there.

In reviewing this case, Dina says that what really helped in this process was, first, a lot of honest, open communication and, second, the relationship which had been built up with Ellen, which allowed her to look at her situation in a very different way:

> Because of the confidence that she had in me, she seemed to be making quite large leaps of progress in her own confidence and to take the

challenge of going into a home ... I'd like to think that the process went well because of a little bit of that extra relationship-building at the outset.

Managing the paperwork

As a community-based home care manager, Amanda carries a caseload of 56 older people. Some are living in residential institutions; others are at home. She prefers the cases where she is able to work with people longer-term:

> I like the long-term ones where I build up that relationship because of how they develop and how you can actually maintain their independence at home and it's their choice.

Amanda likes getting out of the office to see people; she dislikes 'the paperwork', although she understands that it has to be done:

> The downside is the paperwork. It's the paperwork. You spend so much time in the office doing paperwork.

John made a choice to work with older people 5 years ago after working in the children's services. He had enjoyed working with children and families but, like other social workers who have contributed to this book, he had watched experienced staff leaving the service and a series of reorganisations which had resulted in unbearable pressures on front-line social workers. He now feels that his move was a good one, because he has found that older people and their carers are extremely positive about the work he does with them. However, he finds that the growing amount of paperwork and the managerial culture that it reflects detract from what he is able to achieve as a social worker. He describes the way his job has changed in recent years:

> In the 5 years that I have worked with the elderly team, the job has changed enormously. New things have come in – continuing care, unified assessments, fairer charging and with them, there are volumes of paper. When I started my job, the manager said to me, 'It's people before paper', but we now spend an enormous time of our working life behind the desk and the computer. I am not computer literate and when we had a typist I could scrawl a letter and pass it on to her. That's gone now, and it's easier to do it yourself and I do it and I am very slow. We do our own care plans on the computer and it all soaks up and eats into time that we should be spending with people out in the community.

John believes that the social work role with older people is being eroded. As he says, 'We are becoming more like salespeople, going out to people and asking them, "Do you want one of these and one of those?" I think we should be doing more actual social work.' What John means by this is clear:

> When people have lost people after living with them for 40 or 50 years it is a huge void in their lives and I do not think we appreciate that enough now. People need more support than just a hand-rail or home care coming in the morning. They need support emotionally and we do not seem to have time for that any more and that is a frustrating part of our job.

Suzy echoes much of what Dina, Amanda and John have said. She feels that the shift to care management which the 1990 NHS & Community Care Act heralded has been a disservice to those with whom she has been working:

> I do think it is about the change of social work into care management. I think that it is so process-orientated now and paper-orientated that we are losing sight of the person. We don't do counselling any more. If someone loses a partner we are so quick to just fill out a form to say, 'We don't work with the husband any more so we will close the case', leaving Mrs Bloggs hanging in there, grieving. There doesn't seem to be an understanding that we ought to do two to three visits after someone dies.

Suzy moved to a promoted post, in part, because this has a protected caseload, thus allowing her to hold on to some of what she sees as essential for good practice. Now, her workload is more within her control, but there are drawbacks too:

> There are benefits to the job I do now. I get a smaller caseload compared with the rest of the team. I've got 28 community cases and 22 residential and nursing review cases. So I can work in-depth with people and stay involved with them for a long period. I do not like to do an assessment, do a review and then close a case. I can't get used to that system at all. I don't like saying to people who I have been involved with that I'm closing them as a case and they should ring me if they need anything . . . The downside of it is that I am in the office a lot more doing paperwork and developmental work with the team.

Seventy per cent of those who work in Suzy's office are unqualified community care workers, many of whom are nearing retirement. Suzy feels that this explains what she perceives as their lack of interest in training. She says that the arrival of a social work student has been good for her: it has encouraged her to examine her practice again, and to ask the question 'why'.

Risk and protection

Amanda is highly critical of society's attitudes towards older people. She believes strongly that older people should be respected for who they are, and for the lives they have lived, including their experience, in some cases, of two world wars. She asserts: 'They should be seen as valued members of society and in other countries they would be . . .'

As a social worker working with older people in the community, Amanda acknowledges that it is difficult at times to maintain a balance between respecting an older person's wishes and keeping her or him safe. She introduced the story of one older woman with whom she worked to illustrate this point:

> . . . she was barely surviving, but it was her choice. She was safe, she was warm, she was cared for, although her friends and neighbours and family said she needed to be in a home. But she didn't want to be. She would get very agitated at times, she'd call six or seven times in an afternoon, couldn't remember how she got her TV on, or when home care were going to be calling, those sort of things. I just took it in my stride. I got into a routine, I could remember how her telly worked, how to put it on, 'Yes, home care will be there at such and such time' and all that.

While Amanda was off on annual leave, the old lady had a fall and was admitted to hospital. Amanda went to see her and arranged a care package for her coming home. The following night, the old lady fell again, para-medics were called out, and when Amanda went to see her, she had lost her confidence. Amanda tried to arrange for her to spend a few days at a local residential home, but it had no vacancies. She eventually found a space for her in a private residential home. But Amanda found the whole process upsetting because she knew this was not what the old lady had wanted:

> I never thought it would come to this, because it was not what she wanted and I am the perpetrator of this. I had taken her to where she doesn't want to be, because she wants to be at home, and obviously she was born in 1910, she remembers the war time, she remembers the wars and I can remember driving behind her [when she was taken

into care], in tears and I'm thinking, 'Pull yourself together.' I got her there – it was only meant to be for a couple of days but she settled in and she agreed to stay. But I always feel really guilty that I'm the one that put her there; that circumstances had overtaken what I had planned for her and what she had planned for herself. I also felt quite reassured that she needs to be safe and she realised that she needed to be safe . . . I don't think I could have done it any different, I don't know, but I still feel so guilty about it. And yet she settled in lovely and she's looking really well, but at the end of the day I always knew she didn't want to and she did tell me sometimes, 'Oh, I never thought it would come to this.'

Dina also expressed concern that, as a hospital social worker, she is sometimes asked to put pressure on an older person to agree to admission to a nursing home, because doctors and/or family think this is best for him or her. She explains further:

There are times when the hospital wants you to discharge a patient against his or her wishes, and be admitted into a nursing home, and you could do that by getting a signature from the patient, if the family is in compliance. But there are these moral questions, because if you ask a patient whether they want to move into a nursing home – and you are advised that they *need* to do so – and they say, 'No, I've never wanted to go into one – I'd rather die here than go into a nursing home.' And you are told they need to be discharged and you need to get a signature – that's when all your professional, personal, moral and legal issues begin to fuse with each other. That's where my education and confidence are helping me, because I can stand out and say 'No, I think I need to understand this better.'

John also related the story of a time when he had to stand up for an older person.

I was given a referral to go and see a gentleman who was in Bridgend Hospital. The referral said he lived alone and had never received services. He had been abusing alcohol in recent years, he was diabetic and his situation had deteriorated and he had ended up in hospital. I went to see the man on the ward and I was struck by his great command of language. He was an extremely articulate man and I was fascinated by him and I still am – he is such an interesting man. I said we could discuss ways we could help him. He said, 'My son has arranged for me to go to a home near where he lives, 60 miles away.' I asked if this was what he wanted, and he said, 'That's what my son wants.'

John's assessment (supported by his manager) was that the older man was not ready to go into residential care; that he should be given the opportunity to go home. John met the older man's son, and reported his view that social services should not fund a residential place. The son was furious, and put in a complaint about John and his manager. But, as John said, 'I wasn't prepared to budge on the issue. Whether the authority was prepared to budge was another matter, but I wasn't prepared to budge – that was my firm view.' A few days later, the son phoned John to say that he had been thinking about what they had been saying and 'thought possibly it would be a good idea to give dad a chance to go home'. John continues:

> We arranged a large package of care to support the man, in conjunction with the district nurses. That package of care still goes today. I am on the best of terms with the family and the service user greets me warmly every time I go to see him. I thought this was an important moment in my social work career. I advocated for a gentleman for the best reasons and the outcome has been satisfactory. We are now 4 years down the line and he is still home and he is happy and things are going well.

Risk, for older people, is not only about risk from themselves; sometimes they are at risk from others, as Adrian's narrative recounts:

> There was a case I was involved with. A lady was referred by the district nurse; mother and son were living together. The district nurse ... was a bit concerned that the lady was struggling and her son was having to assist her with personal care. I did an assessment and then a couple of weeks later, we had a phone call from the Emergency Duty Team on a Monday morning, and there had been an incident over the weekend where neighbours had called the police because they had heard shouting – the son was shouting at his mother and the Emergency Duty Team had gone out, and the son was found in quite a state and had actually been sectioned and taken to hospital. So when I picked it up that Monday and started digging a bit deeper, it became evident what had really been going on ... from speaking to the neighbours who obviously hadn't said anything up until now, but obviously did now it was all out in the open. So I went along to do an assessment again because the situation had changed; in the community care assessment, we don't just look at the circumstances, we also look at protecting people as well.

LESSONS FOR THE FUTURE

The 2005 White Paper for England, *Our Health, Our Care, Our Say* (Department of Health 2005b), builds on two consultations: the Green Paper *Independence, Wellbeing and Choice* (Department of Health 2005a),[3] and a listening exercise, *Your Health, Your Care, Your Voice*. The White Paper affirms that people with ongoing health and social care needs *want* to live independently; moreover, they want services to be easy to get to, and convenient to use. The White Paper goes on to call for more control for service users and patients, for more flexible, personally tailored services. Those interviewed for this chapter would support the White Paper's aspirations 100 per cent. For example, Dina believes strongly that the person-centred work she has described is at the core of social work's identity:

> What I'd like to see for the future is that social work becomes less task-centred. I believe that the therapeutic and person-centred approach should really be infused again into the social work profession, so that social work can retain its own identity.

Suzy would agree, but is more pessimistic about the future. She believes that social work needs to get back to counselling and away from competencies; she sees registration as good 'if it gives people pride in the profession and may protect vulnerable people'. But she is wary too – 'I don't know that I want to be like a doctor or a barrister because they are in it for themselves. If we are too professional it puts up barriers.'

In reviewing the direction of services for older people in recent years, Lymbery (2005) identifies a shift towards procedural and managerial requirements rather than a more flexible, professional practice. John demonstrates what this means in practice. He said he wants social work to return 'to what it was meant to be'; to the job that he thought he was moving into when he first entered social work. He wants to move away from the situation where you 'go in quickly, arrange things and disappear', and urges the need for time to do therapeutic work, that is, 'supporting people in an emotional way – it's slipped away from that'.

As a user of social services, Brian also believes that social work must hold on to its focus on people. He argues that social work must be more than just a job for people:

> I think the people in social services have to involve themselves in the patient and devote themselves to the patient. Never turn your back – you've got a job and you've got to be seen to be doing something. Devotion to the cause. We've got carers now who do that – the one

girl comes to find me wherever I am and says, 'We're off now – is there anything else you want? See you at tea-time.' These aren't people doing it for money and looking at their watches. They are professionals, centred on the patient. They are respectful.

Annette adds: 'Dignity as well – today's social workers give us that. I don't think anything else can beat it.'

Amanda believes that social workers must not be afraid to make themselves unpopular with their employers. She argues that services must always be centred on what people need:

> As social workers, we must be saying to the powers that be, 'Well, actually, our client doesn't want to go to the day centre, so we need to be looking at other services instead. Perhaps they want to go to the pub 3 days a week . . .' so the services should meet people's needs.

This is the real challenge for social work in providing services for older people: to provide services which are what older people, and those caring for them, need and want, instead of fitting people into existing (and diminishing) services.

ACKNOWLEDGEMENTS

Thanks to Angela Tebboth for helping us make contacts in Wales and Catherine Poulter, Service Manager for Adult Services at Bridgend County Council, for setting up the interviews with social workers and service users.

NOTES

1   A recent study of older people's admission to nursing homes found that decisions were often taken by relatives and professionals, with older people relegated to a 'minor role' (Davies and Nolan 2003).
2   The Social Care Institute for Excellence has produced an online practice guide to assessing the mental health needs of older people. See: http://www.scie.org.uk/publications/practiceguides/bpg2/section02/index.asp
3   The government Green Paper on adult social care, *Independence, Wellbeing and Choice* (Department of Health 2005a), raises key questions on person-centred support, individualised services, choice and control for service users and carers, and resourcing of good practice. The proposals identified to 'deliver this vision' include: wider use of Direct Payments and individual budgets; 'greater focus on preventative services; local government working together with other agencies, particularly the NHS, to ensure a range of provision; the development of new models of service delivery and use of technology' (2005a: 72).

REFERENCES

Arber, S., Davidson, K. and Ginn, J. (eds) (2003) *Gender and Ageing: Changing Roles and Relationships*, Buckingham: Open University Press.

Arber, S. and Ginn, J. (1992) '"In Sickness and in Health": Care-giving, Gender and the Independence of Elderly People', in C. Marsh and S. Arber (eds) *Families and Households. Divisions and Change*, Basingstoke, Hants: Macmillan.

Bytheway, B. (1995) *Ageism*, Buckingham: Open University Press.

Davies, S. and Nolan, M. (2003) 'Making the Best of Things: Relatives' Experiences of Decisions about Care Home Entry', *Ageing and Society*, 23: 429–50.

Department of Health (2005a) *Independence, Wellbeing and Choice. Our Vision for the Future of Social Care for Adults in England*, London: DoH.

Department of Health (2005b) *Our Health, Our Care, Our Say*, White Paper, London: DoH.

Dwyer, S. (2005) 'Older People and Permanent Care', *British Journal of Social Work*, 35(7): 1081–92.

Evandrou, M. and Glaser, K. (2004) 'Family, Work and Quality of Life: Changing Economic and Social Roles through the Lifecourse', *Ageing and Society*, 24(1): 1–21.

Johnstone, J. (2002) 'Taking Care of Later Life: a Matter of Justice?', *British Journal of Social Work*, 32: 739–50.

Kerr, B., Gordon, J., MacDonald, C. and Stalker, K. (2005) *Effective Social Work with Older People*, Research Findings no. 11, December, Edinburgh: Scottish Executive Education Department Research Programme.

Lymbery, M. (2005) *Social Work with Older People*, London: Sage.

Phillipson, C. (2002) 'The Frailty of Old Age', in Davies, M. (ed.) *Blackwell Companion to Social Work*, 2nd edition, Oxford: Blackwell, pp. 58–63.

Ray, M. and Phillips, J. (2002) 'Older People', in Adams, R., Dominelli, L. and Payne, M. (eds) *Critical Practice in Social Work*, Basingstoke, Hants: Palgrave, pp. 199–209.

Chapter 8

Lessons for the future

INTRODUCTION

In reviewing the book as a whole, it is striking how unequivocal service users and carers across the board are about what they want from social workers and social work. They want practitioners to listen to them, to treat them with respect, to see them in the context of their families and communities. They want emotional and material support to enable them to lead independent lives and manage crises and difficulties. They want flexible, responsive and reliable services. Practitioners' stories are also unambiguous about the profession of which they wish to be a part. Most social workers come into social work either out of a desire to help others, or to challenge social injustice. Some practitioners combine both kinds of motivations. What they all enjoy in social work is the opportunity to build relationships with people, to work creatively with them, to make a difference in their lives, and perhaps even in society as a whole. They know that these aspirations sound clichéd, and yet this is what keeps them going in social work.

The book has demonstrated the usefulness of a narrative approach in accessing social work voices 'from the inside'. It gave us so much material that we have only been able to use a fraction of the interview data that we amassed, and some contributors may feel that we have not been able to reflect fully their stories, and indeed their lives. In truth, each chapter could have become a book in its own right, and even then, choices would have had to be made about what to include and what to leave out. We have sought, nevertheless, to be honest throughout about what we were trying to do and to be respectful of the viewpoints and experiences that people shared with us.

This final chapter reviews some of the contributors' main messages about social work and what it needs if it is to thrive, messages which, we believe, should play a part in the debates that are currently informing the future direction of social work in the UK. The chapter draws together what the contributors identified as the characteristics of good social work.

It then considers what organisations should provide in order to promote and sustain good social work. In keeping with the approach which we have adopted throughout the book, we begin each section with the voices of service users and carers.

GOOD SOCIAL WORK

Is responsive

A theme to come out of many accounts is that asking for help is difficult. People usually get in touch with social work agencies because they are desperate; their usual coping mechanisms have broken down and they have nowhere else to turn. Annette and Brian went so far as to say that they only sought help when they realised that they might become the subjects of a newspaper story which reported the deaths of two older people in their home. Given that seeking help is difficult, the response must be timely. When 12-year-old Sarah ran away from home with her younger sister, it was vital that her cry for help was heard and responded to immediately.

The book is full of accounts of people who were at their wits' end by the time social work services were provided. For example, Helen said that she had been 'ringing alarm bells for weeks' and no one seemed to be listening; it took a child protection allegation to get the attention she needed for her husband's mental health problems. Another familiar story is of services being withdrawn because a person seems to be managing OK. Julie found this extremely unhelpful, because she continued to have problems in managing her daughter's behaviour. Some service users had to make a formal complaint in order to get the help they needed. For example, Sian described having no alternative but to make a complaint so that she would be allocated a specialist learning-disabilities social worker, rather than left to deal with whoever was available through the duty system. As a social worker, Michaela confirmed that this was her experience too. She said that new work in her team was only taken on as a result of 'crises or complaints'. The implications of this are hugely negative for service users and for social work, because by the time people get the help they need, 'they are', as she said, 'in a bad way'.

Being responsive in social work also means giving consideration to issues of accessibility. This theme came up in a number of different settings. Helen, as a carer, said that good social workers use language which people will understand, not jargon words, technical terms and initials which are not explained. For Dannielle, accessibility was about geographical setting. When her support services were relocated from the town centre to a large former children's home in the rural area, it was much more difficult for her to access the day-by-day support she needed as a young care-leaver. Whatever the situation, the social work response must be respectful of service users. This is, in part, about acknowledging the strategies they have already tried to manage their difficulties. But it is also about having an appreciation for the intrusion which seeking help inevitably brings. Angela said that she knew that 'the world and his wife' would enter her life when she asked for help, and as a private, independent person, she hated this.

Is about building relationships

A theme reiterated throughout service users' and carers' accounts was that good social work is founded on building relationships with people; only then, Matt argued, are people able to share their difficulties with social workers. This was demonstrated clearly in Mark's relationship with his criminal justice social worker. He said that one of the controls which is keeping him on the 'straight and narrow' is that he does not want to let his social worker down. This suggests a relationship which is more than just professional; it is personal too:

> It helped too that my social worker told me personal things so I told her things – I didn't expect her to tell me things – but she felt relaxed enough to do this with me. It's about relationship, and trust and respect for each other. I feel like I've changed – I won't get in trouble again.

Mark's story shows that relationships are not just one-way. Terri also spoke about this. She said that her social worker, now retired, had been ill, and Terri had been phoning to find out how she was. Her social worker had, in effect, become her 'friend', and their relationship had no endpoint. Many of the social workers also talked about the reciprocal relationships they have with service users and carers. They described how much they had learnt from service users, whom they see as 'experts by experience', with much to teach them about their lives, and about the support they need and want. Barbara made this point in relation to disability services; Niall mirrored this in criminal justice social work. For Kathy, it was quite simple: 'the more you put in, the more you get back'. Colin, a residential worker with young people, added:

> . . . there's not some kind of pixie dust – a magic solution to working with kids, whether it's a risk assessment or a cognitive behavioural programme or whatever – it's actually about relationship, and connection and commitment, and trying to get that message over.

As a hospital social worker faced with the institutional imperative to discharge patients as quickly as possible, Dina argued that her first task is always to build a relationship with the service user. She sees this as the foundation for all future work, and she is prepared to set aside routine expectations of practice to make this happen. In order to build relationships with others, social workers must also be prepared to reflect on who they are and what they are bringing to their social work practice; they must be aware of the impact of themselves on others.

There has been renewed interest in self and identity in recent years, and with this, a reflexive understanding of the person we bring to social work. One service user made a similar point:

> ... you need to know yourself as a social worker – you need to understand who you are, where you've come from, and what you're bringing to the job, otherwise you won't survive personally, and you won't be able to maintain balance in yourself, your personal life and your professional life, and you won't be a good worker.

Is person-centred

There was an awareness in all the accounts in the book that people are different: they have different strengths, motivations, backgrounds, circumstances and, of course, different needs. This means that they are likely to require different kinds of support; there can be no 'one size fits all' in social work services.

The term which was used frequently to describe this was that social work must become 'person-centred': not service-centred or problem-centred, but person-centred. For this to become a reality, a flexible range of services needs to be available for service users and their carers, from individual support, to family work, group work, day centres, respite care and residential care. Moreover, those working in these services must see service users as whole people. For example, Julie was delighted to discover that staff in the family centre to which she was referred were prepared to get to know her for herself, not just as a 'child protection problem'. By not immediately focusing on her drug use, they succeeded in building her confidence so that she was able to tackle her wider problems. Being person-centred may also mean acknowledging that the needs of family members are not necessarily the same as those of the service user. Although Michael's and Harry's children wanted them to be looked after in residential care 'for their own good', their social workers had to recognise that this was not what Michael and Harry wanted for themselves.

Some of the social workers described what being person-centred meant for them. Sarah described how she had encouraged the creativity of a probation client, so that he regularly painted pictures during his visits to her agency for cognitive behavioural group work sessions. Similarly, Gavin's account of running a weekly football match with psychiatric service users and staff demonstrated his firm belief that social work, to be truly person-centred, must be about more than 'talking therapies'. The importance of person-centred social work becomes even more acute when we are thinking about services for children and young people. All the social workers who work with children highlighted the need for social workers to have fun with kids; children in residential care need to have 'normal growing-up activities', urged Mark.

Is about support which is both emotional and practical

It was clear from service users and carers that social work needs to offer both emotional and practical support; that one cannot exist without the other. It was argued that there is little point in offering help with feelings if a person is about to be made homeless; likewise, moving people on to residential care without giving attention to issues such as loss and bereavement is unlikely to be productive in the longer term. Practical support can sometimes provide the avenue for leading into more difficult areas, as Donna outlined. When she was helped to get a nursery place for her daughter, a relationship of trust was built which allowed her to begin to look at other areas of her life, including her drug use. Sian also spoke about the importance of her social worker being prepared to give her practical help:

> I think that social work is about helping people and recognising when people need help. You can dress it up and you can call it all sorts of other things but you must not be too frightened about getting involved in people's lives or being frightened of being accused of being paternalistic sometimes, when actually what people want is help, they don't always want to be empowered or enabled to do the job themselves; they want somebody there who is in 'the know' to help them out of a hole and to recognise the impact that having a job when you have a learning disability can have on a family and on carers, let alone the person with a learning disability.

Ron argued that even in the high-profile field of criminal justice social work, social work must first address the welfare and practical needs of offenders; only once these have been addressed will it be possible to attend to the question of offending behaviour. Ron acknowledged that this may not be what the general public wants, but it is necessary all the same.

Dina also highlighted the extreme poverty experienced by many of the older people with whom she was working. She advised that hospital social work must address the question of material deprivation first, before older people can leave hospital safely. Looking back over her career, Gayle expressed frustration that the resources which children's workers have to access are still inadequate, 30 years after she first entered social work.

Is holistic

Leading on from this, service users asserted that social work must be holistic. Of course, not all the services which people may need to access are social work services. Social work is located in a context of wider services including health, housing and welfare benefits. Jason urged that different services must work together to support people, and that social work has a responsibility to bring these together. He said there must be no repeat of the situation where he and his children were stuck in a very expensive residential unit for a year because no agency was prepared to pay a (relatively small) amount of rent arrears which he owed.

Thinking about this in terms of criminal justice social work, Arlon's recommendation was that we must get back to the idea of community social work, where there is a commitment to improving communities, and, hence, reducing the need for social work in people's lives.

Is about balancing rights, risk and protection

Another predominant theme to emerge in many service users' and carers' accounts is that social work must manage better the complex challenges brought by the need to balance an individual's rights with the possibility of risk and the need to protect the individual and society. Sally and Maggie both acknowledged that, at critical moments in their lives, they had needed to be hospitalised for their own protection. They bore no resentment about this; Sally even said that she would not have been here today if her social worker had not acted quickly on her behalf.

Ellie presented an example of a situation where she had had to balance a woman's need for protection, with the wishes of her family members to keep her at home. She described how she had had to confront her own values in this situation, by questioning what was acceptable behaviour. She acknowledged that, as a mental health social worker, her task was sometimes to be an arbiter of this. The social workers who worked with older people all agreed that their priority was, wherever possible, to facilitate independence; for most service users, that meant keeping them at home in their own environments as long as possible. But this does, at times, imply living with risk. Helen, as a carer, urged that good social work must be prepared to take risks and look at the big picture. Although she said that she understood the pressure on social workers not to get things wrong, she urged that they should not be afraid to make mistakes, because that is how we learn.

Is knowledgeable and evidence-based

It was clear from the service users' and carers' accounts that they want their social workers to be knowledgeable, and to be trained in what they do. They also want their workers to be honest about what they do not know (Maggie and Angela spoke about this from their very different experiences). Beyond this, however, it was the practitioners who had most to say about the need for social work to have an evidence base.

Many illustrated the influence of a 'what works' agenda in social work. They knew about research studies relevant to their area of practice; they wanted their intervention to be as helpful and focused as possible. Yet what came across from all the stories is the unpredictable, complex and highly individual nature of social work. It is clear that what worked for one person in one situation may not have worked for another in another situation. Hence cognitive approaches and counselling were found to be equally successful; likewise a day centre was valued as much as home-based support. Both service users and practitioners indicated that it can take time to see results; it may even be years later that a service user can fully understand the nature of the help which he or she received. This makes accounting for social work help difficult – when do you carry out an evaluation to be sure that it is valid? Perhaps more fundamentally, what questions do you ask? The criminal justice chapter reminded us that 'success', if judged only in terms of a reduction in offending, may be a rare occurrence, but if it is measured in terms of a reduction in the severity of an offence, then we may see more positive results. And what if success is measured in terms of someone's finding and keeping a job, or building and sustaining better relationships with others in their communities? Niall urged that 'we must find things to measure other than statistics'. Meanwhile Mark, currently on probation, said that 'even if only one in 10 people benefit from a service, that's 10 people in every 100'.

Is future-orientated

Many service users talked about how important it is for social work to help them to look to the future; to make realistic plans for their lives, to set goals, to look ahead. In the mental health context, Trish and Sally both said how important this is. As a parent who has accessed social work help, Julie agreed. She felt she had benefited from the opportunity to look at the future in a different way, or as she said, 'to find myself and know where I am going'.

Criminal justice social work is focused on increasing motivations and helping service users to make progress. Fiona reminded us that change from the outside may seem small, but for someone to shift from injecting to smoking heroin is a demonstrable improvement for their health and well-being. Alison argued that to help people to move on, it is necessary to help them identify where they want to be. Ellie described what this meant for her in mental health social work:

> When people go through a horrendous time in their lives and their journey is very painful, and they feel there's no way out and they're coming to see you and you're working, working, and they begin to make sense – and they are working with you on it, and they're bringing work to you because they're making sense – and just to see them walk into the room with their head held up, shoulders back, and you think 'Great – where's the next one?' It doesn't happen that often, really, but that one can make a real difference, when people own the stuff and then they go on their own road.

Is there for the long term

Some of the service users and carers whom we interviewed explained that they are likely to have social work contact for the rest of their lives. There can be no 'quick fix' for some people with disabilities, for some older people and their carers, or for some people with mental health problems. Because of this, service users said they want consistency and long-term support, not to be processed through a succession of short-term social workers. They do not want to have to build relationships afresh every few months, and, perhaps even more critically, they do not want to have to teach their new social workers about Direct Payments, or about any other new policy development.

One of the child and family social workers advised that some adults lack the material, emotional and family resources to be the parents they would like to be, and in these situations, social work needs to be there for the longer haul. All those working in residential child care acknowledged that children in the 'looked-after system' currently have too many social workers, and too many moves; what they need, in contrast, is consistency; someone who will be there for them through the ups and downs of growing up. Some young people did find this long-term connection with a social worker. For example, Sarah said she is still in contact today with someone who had worked at the children's home she entered over 10 years earlier. From her perspective, Arlon confirmed that good criminal justice social work may take time; people's lives do not necessarily turn around within the lifetime of a probation order. Phil agreed; he is continuing to support a young man in the learning disability field even though the young man is now settled and doing well.

THE ORGANISATIONAL CONTEXT OF GOOD SOCIAL WORK

All the contributors recognised that good social work has to have an organisational context that allows it to thrive. Service users and carers said they were most concerned when organisations were unresponsive, or when changes in structure and procedures meant that they had to get to know new systems and new personnel. Many urged that there should be more consistency within organisations and that they should develop better ways of retaining the information that they were continuously asking service users and carers to provide. David's view was that the response which service users get is too often dependent on the individual social worker; he said there needs to be less variability in service delivery.

Most of the detailed comments about what organisations do to help or hinder good social work came, not unexpectedly, from the practitioners. While some had positive things to say about the organisations within which they worked, many also spoke with considerable feeling about the stress and strain of working in organisations that seemed to be in a state of permanent reorganisation. This view was mirrored across all the service sectors represented in this book, and is probably the greatest single source of complaint by the practitioners. Despite this, many practitioners said how much they loved their work. One social worker put it as follows:

> For all the goings-on with social work, I can actually count on one hand the amount of social workers or managers that don't like their job – there is a real commitment there, there's a real expertise, and people are willing to learn as well. I don't think you go into social work just for a vacation – you end up there – you're there for your whole life – if it's for you, you stay there. The vast majority of people that I've met do enjoy it. They'll moan about certain things, but they like their job. I think that speaks volumes, because life would be much easier just to walk away and get a job somewhere else!

What works in social work agencies

Many practitioners praised their colleagues; they said they were working in high-calibre teams with excellent staff. They highlighted the following as essential to enable such teams to exist and even to thrive:

- having managers who understand and value what you are doing and support you in your work;
- a climate in which people can flourish and deliver good social work rather than struggle and fail to deliver on their potential;
- opportunities for staff to work flexible hours (part-time working may be essential to allow some practitioners to balance work and family commitments);
- having students on placement whose learning requires attention and strong role models;
- opportunities for social workers to be promoted while still maintaining contact with practice;
- encouragement for social workers to be creative;
- a hierarchy which is responsive to individual social workers' requests for information;
- systems in place for regular supervision of work;
- time for staff to read and think and exchange ideas;
- opportunities for ongoing training;
- possibilities of carrying out long-term work with service users;
- not being risk-averse – being ready to deal with the unexpected, and prepared to take risks.

What does not work in social work agencies

Structural reorganisation has had a major impact on the working conditions of practitioners. 'Shared futures', 'joint working' and integration of services mean that social workers are increasingly located in large organisations which are not social work departments. Contributors said that they felt that the increasing integration of services holds the potential for both improvements in, and deterioration of, services. Service users look forward to there being better cohesion on the part of those delivering services, as long as this does not lead to any decrease in service-provision. Likewise, social work practitioners believe that they have much to contribute to joint working, in terms of the values and skills they bring, as well as their knowledge. But they are anxious that their profession might become lost in the future; that the social work voice may become drowned out next to the much larger and more powerful voices of education and health.

One practitioner said that structures do not matter to employers so much as doing a good job:

> We've long passed the time when social work was seen as having the answer to a whole set of issues. I would hate to see the people doing the front line work devalued because it needs doing whatever it's called because people need it. It doesn't seem to matter to employers

any more what the people are called that they employ as long as they want to do a good job.

Coping with organisational change has been a major source of stress on the practitioners who took part in this book. Along with change, has come increased paperwork, bureaucracy and new computer systems, all of which have been experienced as having a negative impact on work with service users and their carers. Social workers were unhappy with the computerised systems of recording and assessing which were becoming an increasing part of their lives. They told us that they came into the profession because they wanted to work with people, not pieces of paper or machines. They also want to do more than just carry out assessments, rewarding as this can be. They want to intervene, to see things through, to walk alongside people, to deliver a service. This was demonstrated by one practitioner who said she wanted to be 'a social worker, not a technician'.

Niall spoke passionately about the importance of keeping motivation high in social work. He was unapologetic about the need to give attention to this in spite of other pressures:

> You can't do this work if you are not motivated. It's how you main-
> tain that motivation, and the things that kill it. Sometimes the
> bureaucracy of agencies can kill the whole approach to working with
> people. I know there's a need for it, but it can be a case of the tail
> wagging the dog, and sometimes I have to remind my colleagues of
> that. We're here to provide a service. I'm not working for the HR
> [Human Resources] department or the finance department – I'm here
> to provide a service to clients, and that's the way it's going to be.
> And I'm not here to keep my manager in a job either.

We have argued that social work is fundamentally about being along-side people in their lives. Whatever assessment forms are being completed, reports being written, or packages of care being devised, we must be prepared to give priority to looking again at how we use ourselves in a critical and reflexive way. Moreover, people's lives are complex, and their problems likewise; if this were not the case, they would manage without social workers. This complexity brings with it a mixture of emotional, physical, psychological, environmental, social and even spiritual concerns. Social workers need support to do this job well, through supervision and through opportunities for reflection and further learning. Furthermore, agencies must become learning organisations, in which practitioners can be encouraged to embrace new ideas and challenges, and move to new positions where they might be re-energised and renew their commitment to the profession.

LOOKING AHEAD

We stated at the beginning of this book that social work is changing: its structures, organisation and professional position are all being renegotiated as we write. Its central function does not, however, change. In thinking about social work in the future, a theme which stands out from the interviews is best summed up by the practitioner who said that she felt that social work had been, to date, 'a quiet profession'. In this, she reflected a view expressed by many of those whom we interviewed, that social work needs to stand up and be counted; we need to be much clearer about what social work can, and cannot, offer; we need to be willing to contribute to public debates about issues as diverse as offending and the impact of poverty on the lives of those using social work services. A criminal justice social worker put it this way:

> Social work is very susceptible to government wish lists about what they want done, whether this is offenders, or mentally disordered people, reducing residential care, etc. . . . As a profession, we need to be more confident about what we can offer, and more certain about what we cannot offer – that would be my wish for us.

We hope that this book, in its own way, will make a contribution to this process. We end with the voice of Sarah, a care-leaver who is about to begin her social work degree programme:

> I'm really passionate about social work – we *can* make a difference and inform practice and legislation. I know the difference social services made in my life, and I think I could do it, and do it really well. I know there's a lot of regulations and a lot of pressure – but I really want to do it and think that I can make a difference.

Index